D1523451

CLINIMETRICS

Clinimetrics

Alvan R. Feinstein, M.D.

Yale University Press
New Haven and London

Published with assistance from the Louis Effingham deForest Memorial Fund.

Designed by James J. Johnson and set in Times Roman type by Delmas. Printed in the United States of America by Murray Printing Company, Westford, Mass.

Library of Congress Cataloging-in-Publication Data

Feinstein, Alvan R., 1925–
  Clinimetrics.

  Bibliography: p.
  Includes index.
  1. Diagnosis—Decision making. 2. Diagnosis—
Measurement. 3. Medicine, Clinical—Decision making.
I. Title. [DNLM: 1. Epidemiologic Methods.
2. Evaluation Studies. 3. Research—methods.
WA 950 F299ca]
RC71.3.F44   1987   616.07′5   86–28241
ISBN 0–300–03806–2 (alk. paper)

The paper in this book meets the guidelines for permanence and durability of the Committee on Production Guidelines for Book Longevity of the Council on Library Resources.

10 9 8 7 6 5 4 3 2 1

Contents

*To students, colleagues, and friends
who stimulate the search for knowledge
and who nurture the searchers*

Preface

This book has been gestating for more than twenty years, ever since I began writing about clinical judgment in patient care.[38] My original discussions were devoted to judgment as an artful science with which clinicians arrange and interpret the data used in clinical decisions. In subsequent writing, I extensively discussed the scientific architecture[54] and statistical procedures[47] used for the arrangements and interpretations. I did not, however, give much emphasis to the methods of formulating the basic clinical information on which all the other activities depended.

I deliberately left this topic to be considered at a later date because I knew a suitable discussion would require some entirely new kinds of thinking. The type of measurement that occurs when raw information is assembled in groups, counted, compared, and statistically analyzed is very different from the measurement that creates the raw information. In the first type of thinking, we might decide what attributes to use in selecting a group of patients and we might choose a mean, median, or some other statistic to summarize their individual ratings of 1+, 2+, 3+, or 4+ for severity of illness. The second type of thinking, however, involves a different set of decisions. We would have to determine what is meant by "severity of illness" and what criteria are used to rate each category as 1+, 2+, 3+, or 4+.

Despite the obvious importance of clinical information, it has not received the intellectually vigorous formal consideration that is given in modern medicine to the paraclinical data obtained with laboratory tests, cytology, biopsy, radiographic imaging, and other technologic procedures. Someone who wants to measure a chemical constituent of the human body can readily find appropriate directions for doing so. The directions will indicate standard methods for setting up the laboratory, checking the reagents, calibrating the equipment, doing the procedure, evaluating the results, and removing any flaws revealed during the evaluations. These methods of quality control have been well established; and the laboratory data are readily accepted as "hard" information that can be scientifically trusted.

No established system of quality control exists, however, for analogous measurements of the human and clinical phenomena that occur in patient care. Appraisals of the existence of a disease, magnitude of a symptom, severity of an illness, or effects of a disability are seldom regarded as measurements, and standard procedures have not been developed for making, checking, evaluating, or improving the appraisals. In the absence of a formal set of methods and standards, the information is usually regarded as too "soft" to receive scientific credibility. Consequently, important human and clinical phenomena are regularly omitted when patient care is recorded in compu- terized "data banks" or analyzed in statistical comparisons of therapy. The phenomena are omitted either because they lack formal expressions to identify them or because the available expressions are regarded as scien- tifically unacceptable.

To give clinical information the attention it warrants, I wanted to develop a counterpart of the strategies, principles, and procedures that are used in creating methods and standards for other forms of measurement. The counterpart would have to be a counterpart, not a resemblance, because of the many fundamental differences between clinical and laboratory forms of measurement. Clinical indexes consist of arbitrary categories and ratings; the described phenomena are much more complex and diverse than the relatively simpler entities cited with laboratory dimensions; and the same clinical phenomenon may have to be measured differently for different purposes. For example, we might need four different rating scales for congestive heart failure if the ratings are used (1) to note the existence of the failure, (2) to grade its relative magnitude, (3) to predict its prognosis, and (4) to choose its treatment. Beyond all these distinctions, clinical ratings often have to be constructed and evaluated with principles that are strikingly different from those used in conventional forms of laboratory measurement. For example, the concepts of *reproducibility* and *accuracy* for laboratory data often cannot be applied to clinical rating scales and often are replaced by different concepts, called *reliability* and *validity*.

In thinking about how the work should be developed, I knew that some of the ideas could come entirely from armchair contemplation, but I wanted the main thoughts to emerge from the pragmatic reality of the clinical activities. To provide the raw material for that reality, I had collected several thousand reprints and other publications that contained clinical indexes and rating scales. From a review and appraisal of that material, the ideas, classifications, and principles could be developed on a solid clinical basis.

What was missing, however, was the time and help with which to do that massive review and appraisal. This opportunity was made available several years ago by a research grant from the Commonwealth Fund. If a rating scale existed for gratitude, I would use its highest score to express my thanks to Margaret E. Mahoney, President, and Thomas W. Moloney, Vice President of the Commonwealth Fund, for their perception of the value of this type of research, and for their enthusiastic support.

Although sustenance from the Commonwealth Fund was the sine qua non for this research, some of my concomitant or ancillary activities were also aided by other sources, whose support I want to acknowledge gratefully. Those sources were the Robert Wood Johnson Foundation (Grant 6309), the Andrew W. Mellon Foundation, and the Cooperative Studies Program Coordinating Center of the West Haven Veterans Administration Hospital.

In planning the research, I at first thought that my colleagues and I would engage in work analogous to draining a swamp. We would go through those thousands of publications, see what was there, classify it appropriately, arrive at some general principles and standards, and then prepare an annotated compendium of clinimetric indexes for each condition we encountered. The annotated compendium would resemble the evaluations of products that often appear in magazines such as *Consumer Reports.* We would tabulate all the clinical indexes (or rating scales) available for each clinical condition, and each index would be accompanied by succinct comments about its applicability and scientific quality. I even thought we might be able to designate certain indexes as a "best buy."

After we started the research and got into the swamp, however, I realized that my original plans and hopes were naive. The state of the art in clinical indexes had good news and bad news that made certain things much better and others much worse than I had expected. The number of indexes we found was much larger than I had anticipated. Despite the general scientific prejudice against soft data, clinicians had often gone ahead and created indexes for the soft phenomena investigated in their research. In some fields, a plethora of indexes had been developed. For example, more than 150 indexes had been published for patients with peptic ulcer disease and more than 225 for locomotor disease. The good news, therefore, was that clinical investigators had been much more productive than I expected in formulating clinical indexes.

The bad news, however, came from this same productivity. Most of the indexes had been developed in an ad hoc or laissez-faire manner. They had been conceived, formulated, and applied directly in clinical trials or other studies without being checked for observer variability, accuracy, or other features of quality in scientific measurement. Many other indexes were essentially redundant, containing minor variations on a previous index whose existence the authors had not discovered when they proposed their "new" one. Thus, an old existing rating scale for citing a certain discomfort as **none, slight, moderate, severe** might have been ignored when investigators proposed a new rating scale of **none, mild, moderate, severe.**

The bad news and good news led to substantial changes in the research plans. Because of the bad news—i.e., the investigators had seldom reported an evaluation of scientific quality for the indexes—we had to abandon the idea of an annotated compendium. The information needed for the annotations was seldom available. Because of the good news—i.e., so many different indexes had been developed—we had to abandon the idea of preparing a complete compendium that would appear in a single book. We had neither the time nor the large research staff that would be needed to organize the entire immense array of diverse information that had been cited in clinical indexes. Even if we had the time and personnel to do so, however, the book would have been enormous and would be unwieldy both to write and to read.

Accordingly, we changed our goals. Instead of assembling a single huge compendium of indexes for all clinical conditions, we selected a few conditions for which we would prepare small compendia to be published separately in appropriate medical journals. The results could serve as a stimulus or prototype for other people who might later want to use the same approach for other conditions. In accordance with this goal, we have already published an annotated commentary on indexes of disability,[61] and we are currently preparing the text of compendia for indexes dealing with peptic ulcer disease, locomotor disease,[63] and congestive heart failure.[62]

Our other goal is accomplished with this book. Its aim is to describe a set of methods, strategies, and principles for constructing and evaluating clinimetric indexes. The absence of any *clinical* standards for this activity was the most striking thing that emerged from our review of the vast literature. In other types of measurement in nonclinical fields, statistical, psychometric, and sociometric standards have been established by workers in those fields and are appropriate for the corresponding statistical or psychosocial goals. But no one has stated the goals of clinical measurement, recognized the occasional or frequent conflict between the clinical goals and the statistical-psychosocial goals, identified the problems that might arise from the conflicts, or proposed ways of resolving the problems. Many of the discussions in this book (particularly Chapter 10 on the evaluation of sensibility) are intended to remedy this defect. The discussions can be helpful to clinicians themselves and also to statistical or psychosocial collaborators who want to know more about the clinician's ethos in measurement.

In addition to the problem of working without a specified set of standards and goals, clinicians have also had difficulty in understanding the concepts, methods, and nomenclature of their collaborating statistical or psychosocial consultants. Clinicians are often confused by the statistical tactics used to form or evaluate clinical indexes, and are generally baffled by the scientifically unfamiliar and conceptually diverse ways in which psychosocial researchers use such terms as *reliability* and *validity*. To help clinicians understand what is needed for effective research or collaboration, I have tried to offer what I hope will be a reasonably clear explanation of the statistical and psychosocial ideas. The explanations appear mainly in Chapters 8, 9, 11, and 12. Another distinctive feature of the book is the taxonomy presented in Chapter 14. If you want to prepare a compendium of clinical indexes for a particular clinical condition, this scheme of classification offers a useful pattern for the arrangement.

The people who helped in the research had a challenging but often tedious job. They had to read through the published material, find the clinical indexes, excerpt the appropriate contents and comments, and pursue the literature further when pertinent. As the chief research lieutenant in those activities, Carolyn K. Wells was a constant source of perception and patience. Although several research assistants participated at various times, the most valuable contributions came (in alphabetical order) from Bruce R. Josephy, Cynthia M. Joyce, and Cindy Sweberg. I thank them all for their help and talent.

For consultative advice in the interpretation of psychosocial indexes, I thank John J. Norcini, Director of Psychometrics for the American Board of Internal Medicine, and James A. Wells, of the Departments of Sociology and Epidemiology at Yale University. I also thank James F. Jekel, Professor of Epidemiology and Public Health at Yale, whose lectures on psychosocial indexes were a valuable introduction for me.

My last word of thanks is for the devoted work of Mary B. Newbury who, sometimes aided by Angela C. Voss, splendidly carried out the task of converting the hand-written manuscript into word-processed text.

ALVAN R. FEINSTEIN
New Haven, Connecticut

Chapter 1

Introduction

Like Molière's bourgeois gentleman who was astonished to discover that he spoke in prose, patients and clinicians may not realize that they constantly communicate with clinimetric indexes. Patients use clinimetric forms of measurement when they say they have *severe* pain, a *slight* headache, a *large gain* in weight, or a *great improvement* in appetite. Clinicians frequently use these same kinds of expressions, but also employ individual clinimetric ratings that are cited in such terms as *2+ sick, Apgar 8, TNM Stage III*, or *New York Heart Association Functional Class IV*.

Although each of the foregoing italicized phrases describes the relative magnitude of a particular entity, the expressions are seldom regarded as acts of measurement. Instead, the expressions are usually attributed to an artful process of personal evaluation and judgment. Many patients and clinicians may even become intensely distressed by the idea that the "art" produces a "measurement" and that the process can be given so formidable a name as *clinimetrics*.[51,60] The distress probably arises from the fear that formal clinimetric attention to these acts of measurement may threaten the few remaining features of humanistic clinical art that have managed to survive the technologic transformations of modern medical science.

The purpose of the proposed clinimetric activities, however, is to improve clinical art, not to impair it. In the current climate of technology and science, the artful citation of important human phenomena is regarded as soft data. These soft citations are used for all the distresses, discomforts, and other sensations that constitute clinical symptoms, as well as for the anxiety, gratification, love, hate, sorrow, joy, and other important human reactions that occur in both sickness and health. Nevertheless, when competing scientifically with the hard data derived from technologic forms of measurement, the soft clinical information may be overlooked or deliberately ignored in the statistics assembled to evaluate the risks, benefits, or other accomplishments of modern medicine. Because the important clinical and human phenomena are either undescribed, i.e., "unmeasured," or excluded from formal consideration, the data used for evaluating patient care become dehumanized. The crucial, uniquely human information has been omitted from the analyses.

These omissions produce major flaws in the art and science of patient care, as well as in the education of clinicians. In clinical art, the clinical information indicates distinctly human characteristics that differentiate people from animals, tissues, or molecules. If we say that cardiac size became smaller, that cardiac rhythm became normal, and that certain enzyme values were lowered, the description could pertain to a rat, a dog, or a person. But if we say that chest pain disappeared, that the patient was able to return to work, and that the family was pleased, we have given a human account of human feelings and observations.

In clinical science, the clinical data act as harbingers of prognosis, determinants of therapy, and identifiers of the "material" subjected to the technologic and other interventions of modern medicine. The clinical information helps denote the severity of illness used in estimating prognosis, the changes of pain and other symptoms that lead to alterations in therapy, and the subgroups of patients, with different kinds of clinical manifestations, who are likely to respond well or poorly to different types of treatment. If the cogent clinical information is omitted, the groups of patients under appraisal may seem similar because they all have the same disease, but the groups may be highly diverse in their clinical composition and clinical outcomes. The results appraised in these heterogeneous mixtures may then have all the scientific credentials of hard data while lacking the basic scientific requirements for reproducible, precise specification of the objects under investigation.

In medical education, we cannot effectively teach the principles and practice of clinical art if we do not identify the principles or demonstrate their usage. They might be learned—like all other features of clinical care—from protracted, thoughtful experience; but the role of formal education is to help ease the younger generation's path in learning the wisdom of the past, while avoiding the many errors that may have led to the wisdom. For clinical art to be taught effectively to modern students, therefore, the teaching cannot depend merely on undocumented experience and unspecified judgment. The teachers will have to do more than give a nebulous discussion of art; they will have to identify what they are talking about.

As for the fear that clinimetric activities will impair clinical art, a great many reassuring observations can be offered. The art of personal care for patients has usually been advanced rather than hampered by the attention needed to rate a newborn baby's Apgar score, a cancer patient's TNM Stage, a cardiac patient's functional class, or any patient's relative magnitude of pain, headache, weight gain, improvement in appetite, anxiety, distress, or satisfaction. The focus on the patient as a person is surely strengthened when specific consideration and analysis must be given to data that come directly from personal conversation, rather than from the patient's blood, urine, feces, tissues, cells, films, or electrographic tracings.

Regardless of the merits of these arguments, however, clinimetric activities warrant formal attention because they are there. At least 43 different indexes have been developed for classifying a patient's functional disability in the self-care and mobility that are called "activities of daily living."[61] The status of patients with congestive heart failure has been cited with 52 different forms of clinical expression.[62] At least 230 rating scales have been proposed for describing the condition of patients with arthritis and other impairments in locomotion.[63]

In almost every disease, condition, or ailment that receives attention in modern medicine, methods have been developed for describing or rating the observed clinical phenomena. The expressions may or may not be formal, standardized, generally accepted, or frequently used—but their very existence indicates that the process of clinimetric measurement is already well established. What the process lacks, however, is a name, a set of well-defined principles and strategies, and an intellectual home. The purpose of these essays is to provide that home, to label it as *clinimetrics,* and to discuss its goals and methods.

During the advances of the past century, enormous efforts have been made to improve the quality of different types of medical information. Well-established systems of taxonomy have been developed to provide consistent categories of classification for *demographic data,* referring to such entities as age, gender, race, religion, and occupation; for *therapeutic-agent data,* referring to pharmaceutical substances, surgical procedures, and other acts of treatment; and for *administrative data,* such as hospital location, type of medical insurance, and mechanisms of payment. For the *paraclinical data* that emerge from such procedures as laboratory tests, microbiology, radiologic imaging, microscopic pathology, and electrographic tracings, special methods have been created to calibrate instruments, standardize procedures, and provide "quality control" in the measurement process.

A specific set of principles and strategies has not yet been developed, however, for the distinctively *clinical data* that emerge from the clinician's work in directly examining patients and in reasoning with the information thereby obtained. There are no standard methods, rules, or taxonomic systems for the clinical processes with which clinicians note symptoms and physical signs, and for the additional information created with diagnostic, prognostic, therapeutic, and other clinical decisions.

During the past two decades, substantial attention has been given to the intellectual mechanisms of clinical decisions. The mechanisms have been described with judgmental formulations, algorithms, flow charts, and a variety of mathematical models. At a more fundamental level of observation and reporting, however, relatively little attention has been given to the quality of the basic clinical information that is processed with these mechanisms. Despite the various formal methods that have been proposed for a clinician's job in reasoning with the acquired data, a distinctive discipline has not been developed for the observations, descriptions, and classifications that constitute the basic measurement process in acquiring the data.

In many other fields of science and the humanities, a *-metry* or *-metrics* suffix has been used to indicate these fundamental acts of mensuration. The first of the hybrid terms, *biometry,* was used by Sir Francis Galton almost a century ago for the domain formed when statistical quantification was joined to biologic sagacity. Later on, as biometry became too mathematical or too inhospitable to a larger scope of biology, three new *-metric* domains were developed. *Anthropometry* was established by anthropologists to deal with gross physical measurements of the human body. *Sociometry* was established by sociologists to deal with rating scales and other methods of measuring cultural, familial, and social phenomena. And *psychometrics* became the home for two different activities: the indexes developed to describe personal and interpersonal behavior, and the work done by specialists in educational testing and examination.

Beyond these biologic activities, the *-metric* domains have subsequently been extended into *econometrics,* as a site for the mathematical models and analyses of economists; *technometrics,* for the work of engineers; *cliometrics* (named after Clio, the muse of history), for the work of historians or political scientists; and *bibliometrics,* for the work of librarians and other information specialists.

The idea and name of *clinimetrics,* therefore, are neither new nor novel. A large family of *-metric* siblings has been awaiting the arrival of *clinimetrics* and probably wondering why it took clinicians so long to get there.

In a complete definition, *clinimetrics* could be regarded as the measurement of clinical phenomena, but the idea of measurement can be divided into two different types of activity. In one form of measurement, which might be called *mensuration,* we acquire and label the basic raw data for the observed phenomena. Mensuration is what we do when we measure individual persons to create such variables and raw data as *birthplace:* **Connecticut;** *gender:* **female;** *age* (in years): **42;** and *functional status:* **Grade 4.**

The other type of measurement might be called *quantification.* It consists of collecting raw data into a group, summarizing the contents of the group, and sometimes comparing the contents of two or more groups. With quantification, we might say that in a particular group of 57 persons, 81% of the members were born in Connecticut, 56% were women, the mean age was 46.2 years, and the median functional status was Grade 3. With a further act of quantification, we might compare this group with a second group of people to reach the conclusion that the second group was relatively older or younger, in better or worse functional status, with relatively more men or women, etc.

During the past eighteen years, the name *clinical epidemiology* has often been used for the second type of measurement, involving quantification and quantified comparisons of clinical phenomena.[54] To distinguish the two forms of measurement, *clinimetrics* will therefore be confined here to the activities in mensuration. (Alternatively, clinical epidemiology could be regarded as a subset of clinimetrics, or clinimetrics as a subset of clinical epidemiology.)

With this constraint, *clinimetrics* can be defined as the domain concerned with indexes, rating scales, and other expressions that are used to describe or measure symptoms, physical signs, and other distinctly clinical phenomena in clinical medicine. The purpose of this book is to propose *clinimetrics* as the name and intellectual home for these activities in clinical mensuration, and to help give them a specific intellectual discipline with well-defined procedures and standards.

Chapter 2

Nomenclature and Functional Classification of Clinimetric Indexes

When a clinician says that a patient has "acute myocardial infarction, with severe chest pain and moderate congestive heart failure," the statement contains four different clinimetric measurements. **Myocardial infarction** is a diagnostic name that measures the existence of a particular disease; **acute** is a measurement of time; **severe** and **moderate** measure the grades of magnitude or severity for a particular clinical condition. These expressions are seldom regarded as measurements because most people think of measurement as an activity that produces dimensional numbers, not verbal categories. To describe height, we might not regard **tall** as a measurement, although **201 cm** would be immediately accepted. For describing weight, **fat** would be deemed an impression, but **149 kg** would be a measurement.

This dimensional constraint on the idea of measurement is easy to maintain whenever a suitable technologic device has been developed to provide the desired numerical value, but the constraint is inappropriate for the many aspects of biology in which the observed substances or phenomena are measured with words, rather than numbers. The verbal measurements include all the distinctions that identify different species of animals, different types of blood cells, different patterns of chromosomes, and the various mitochondria, microtubules, and organelles seen with electron microscopy. When the observed object is a patient, the phenomena that are most distinctive of human life and usually most important for individual persons must be described with verbal expressions. As noted earlier, such phenomena include the distresses and discomforts that are important clinical entities, as well as such associated human reactions as anxiety, fear, love, hate, sorrow, satisfaction, and joy.

6

The effort to identify and specify these clinically vital human phenomena is a task in clinimetric measurement.[53] The measurements can be expressed in unranked verbal categories, such as **myocardial infarction;** in ranked categorical grades, such as **acute, moderate,** or **severe;** in arbitrary numerical ratings, such as **1+** or **4+**; or in any other format that will be suitable and effective. As a general name for these different mechanisms and products of measurement, we can use the term *index.*

An index refers to a class of information that is expressed in a scale of categories. In mathematical parlance, the word *variable* is also used to denote a class of information that is expressed in a scale of categories. Any index can be regarded as a variable, or vice versa. Many clinimetric indexes, however, are created as a combination of several different variables. To show this distinction, the word **variable** will often be reserved here for the elemental components, and **index** will usually be applied to the composite expression. For example, in describing summer weather, *temperature* and *humidity* are each variables, but they are sometimes combined into a composite expression called the *temperature-humidity index.* In winter weather, temperature and wind speed may be combined into a composite index called the *wind-chill factor.* Since clinimetric indexes are not always composite, we can allow for both the simple and the more complex expressions if we regard an index as a class of information expressed in a scale of arbitrarily created categories.

The class of information can be the existence of a particular diagnosis (cited as **present** or **absent**), the grade of severity of a particular condition (cited as **1+, 2+, 3+,** or **4+**), a prediction of prognosis (cited as **excellent, good, fair,** or **poor**), or any other clinical phenomenon that warrants attention, description, and specification.

For example, *age in years* is an index (or variable) expressed in a scale such as **1, 2,..., 30, 30,..., 99,....** The chemical measurements of such entities as *sodium, potassium,* or *cholesterol* are variables (or indexes) expressed in scales of dimensional concentration such as **mg/dl.** *Gender* is an index (or variable) usually expressed in a scale of **male** or **female.** In the examples just cited, each index (or variable) seemed to have an obviously familiar, natural, or customary scale of expression. For many clinimetric indexes, however, the scales of expression are unfamiliar, because they have been arbitrarily created for the particular phenomenon that is being described, or the expression that emerges contains a composite rating for several component entities.

Clinimetric indexes can cite the absence, presence, or degree of magnitude for relatively simple clinical entities, such as pain, discomfort, or distress. The indexes can also reflect complex clinical decisions in making diagnoses, grading severity, estimating prognosis, choosing treatment, or evaluating post-therapeutic accomplishment. Examples of four complex clinimetric indexes are shown in Tables 2.1 to 2.4. The indexes are the New York Heart Association classification of cardiac disability (Table 2.1),[24] the Apgar Score for the condition of a newborn baby (Table 2.2),[5] the Killip classification of severity in acute myocardial infarction (Table 2.3),[101] and the Jones Criteria for diagnosis of acute rheumatic fever (Table 2.4).[3] Other examples of complex clinimetric indexes are the Glasgow coma scale,[150] the Lansbury index of "activity" in rheumatoid arthritis,[110] and the TNM staging system for cancer.[4]

This chapter is devoted to the nomenclature and general function of clinimetric indexes.

2.1. **Nomenclature of Clinimetric Indexes**

Clinimetric indexes can readily be found in the collections of published data that summarize the results of clinical research. The indexes regularly appear in any descriptive account of any patient, but they become particularly evident whenever the results for a group of patients are given a quantitative summary. The indexes that have received these quantitative summaries appear as labels for the rows and columns of tables, as the names entered on the horizontal and vertical axes of graphs, and in the titles given to the expressions of means, medians, rates, or other statistical "reductions" of data. Although any of the different types of medical data can be used for the statistical summaries, and although all the data can be included in the total scope of clinimetrics, clinimetric activity is specifically concerned with indexes that contain distinctly clinical forms of data.

Clinimetric indexes are not always called *indexes.* They may be designated as *scales, scores, factors, stages, classes, ratings, systems,* or *criteria* rather than *indexes.* The titles of clinimetric indexes are often labeled eponymically when the originator's name is applied by subsequent users. This manner of christening was applied for previously mentioned indexes that now commemorate Apgar,[5] Killip,[101] and Jones,[3] and for other indexes that refer to Rose,[137] Peel,[130] and Norris.[126] An eponym need not be personal: the Glasgow Coma Scale[150] is named for the city where it was developed, and the TNM Staging System for cancer[4] is an acronymic eponym using the first letters of the tumor, nodes, and metastases that are the component variables of the index.

In many other instances, however, a clinimetric index has no eponymic title. Sometimes it is labeled generically, e.g. Sickness Impact Profile,[8] and sometimes the index has no name at all. It may have been used once during a particular study and then never employed again; or the originator and subsequent users may not have given it a title.

Table 2.1. Outline of New York Heart Association Functional Classification

Class I	Patients with cardiac disease but without resulting limitations of physical activity. Ordinary physical activity does not cause undue fatigue, palpitation, dyspnea, or anginal pain.
Class II	Patients with cardiac disease resulting in slight limitation of physical activity. They are comfortable at rest. Ordinary physical activity results in fatigue, palpitation, dyspnea, or anginal pain.
Class III	Patients with cardiac disease resulting in marked limitation of physical activity. They are comfortable at rest. Less than ordinary physical activity causes fatigue, palpitation, dyspnea, or anginal pain.
Class IV	Patients with cardiac disease resulting in inability to carry on any physical activity without discomfort. Symptoms of cardiac insufficiency or of the anginal syndrome may be present even at rest. If any physical activity is undertaken, discomfort is increased.

Source: The Criteria Committee of the New York Heart Association, Inc., *Diseases of the Heart and Blood Vessels: Nomenclature and Criteria for Diagnosis,* 6th ed. (Boston: Little, Brown, 1964).
This classification, although still commonly used, has not appeared in subsequent editions of this publication.

Table 2.2. Outline of the Apgar Score for Rating Clinical Condition of a Newborn Baby

	Score		
Variable	*0*	*1*	*2*
Color	Blue; Pale	Body Pink; Extremities Blue	All Pink
Heart rate	Absent	<100	>100
Respiration	Absent	Irregular; Slow	Good, Crying
Reflex response to nose catheter	None	Grimace	Sneeze; Cough
Muscle tone	Limp	Some Flexion of Extremities	Active

Source: V. Apgar, "Proposal for a new method of evaluation of the newborn infant," *Anesth. Anal.* 1953;32:260–7.

Table 2.3. Outline of the Killip Classification for Rating Severity of Myocardial Derangement in Acute Myocardial Infarction

A. *No heart failure*	No clinical signs of cardiac decompensation.
B. *Heart failure*	Diagnostic criteria include rales, S_3 gallop, and venous hypertension.
C. *Severe heart failure*	Frank pulmonary edema.
D. *Cardiogenic shock*	Signs include hypotension (systolic pressure of 90 mm Hg or less) and evidence of peripheral vasoconstriction such as oliguria, cyanosis, and diaphoresis. Heart failure, often with pulmonary edema, has also been present in the majority of these patients.

Source: T. Killip and J. T. Kimball, "Treatment of Myocardial Infarction in a Coronary Care Unit: A Two Year Experience with 250 Patients," *Am. J. Cardiol.* 1967;20:457–64.

Table 2.4. Outline of the Modified Jones Criteria for Diagnosis of Acute Rheumatic Fever

Major Manifestations	*Minor Manifestations*
Carditis	Previous rheumatic fever or rheumatic heart disease
Arthritis	Arthralgia
Chorea	Fever
Erythema marginatum	Acute phase reactions (elevated erythrocyte sedimentation rate, C-reactive protein, or white blood count)
Subcutaneous nodules	Prolonged P-R interval

Diagnosis requires two major elements *or* the combination of one major and two minor elements, together with culture or antibody evidence of preceding Group A streptococcal infection.

Source: G. H. Stollerman, M. Markowitz, A. Taranta, L. W. Wanamaker, and R. Whittemore, "Jones Criteria (Revised) for Guidance in the Diagnosis of Rheumatic Fever," *Circulation* 1965;32:664–8.
These criteria are substantially unchanged in their latest revision, which appeared in *Circulation* 1984;69:204A–8A.

2.2.   Axes of Classification for Clinimetric Indexes

Just as library books can be classified in many different ways—according to author, subject matter, date of publication, color, or size—clinimetric indexes can be catalogued according to various fundamental attributes of their structure and function. The structural attributes include the selected evidence, component parts, mode of combination, and output scale that are inherent in the construction of the index. The functional attributes include the role of the indexes in clinical decisions, statistical analyses, and the architectural arrangements of clinical research.

Like the subject matter of a library book, the clinical function of an index is its most important attribute. Although clinimetric indexes play vital roles in the architectural plan of research projects and in the statistical citation of results, the primary distinction of an index is in its clinical usage. After the index serves its basic clinical role, the data become transferred to a statistical role, which is determined by the architectural arrangement of the research.

The discussion and classification of these roles may seem to be an unexciting, sterile exercise in taxonomy, but the exercise itself has crucial importance in the evaluation of indexes. If we want to determine how well an index does its job, we need first to have a clear idea of the jobs it can be assigned to do.

2.3.   Clinical Functions

Like other forms of data, clinimetric indexes are used to describe conditions, note changes, make predictions, and choose interventions. The subdivisions of these four basic functions create many distinctive roles for the indexes.

2.3.1.   STATUS INDEXES

A status index identifies the state of a particular entity at a single point in time. The index can serve as a "noun," denoting the presence or absence of the entity; or as an "adjective," denoting the magnitude, degree, or other characteristic of an existing entity. For example, the *Jones Diagnostic Criteria* act as a noun, indicating the existence of rheumatic fever; the *TNM Stage* is an adjective, describing the anatomic extensiveness of a cancer. An adjective index can be converted into a noun if one or more of the categories is used to denote the existence of a particular group of people. Thus, although often used as an adjective, *TNM Stage* becomes a noun in a study restricted to patients who are in **TNM Stage III.** Conversely, a noun index can serve as an adjective when it becomes a member of a set of descriptive categories for a delineated group of people. Thus, the diagnostic criteria for rheumatic fever, for lupus erythematosus, for rheumatoid arthritis, or for other ailments become adjectives in an index such as *type of co-existing disease.*

The main clinical use of status indexes is to identify the diagnoses of disease, ratings of clinical conditions, and types of therapeutic agents discussed in the sections that follow.

2.3.1.1. *Diagnostic Criteria*

A fundamental act of clinical reasoning is the diagnosis of a disease. This act requires two separate processes of classification. The first process, which is sometimes called *nosology* or *nosography,* is an act of pure taxonomy. It produces an organized catalog of the entities that can be regarded as diseases. These entities are usually first encountered during medical education in histopathology, but the diseases include many ailments (such as hyperventilation syndrome and schizophrenia) that are not manifested morphologically; and the contents of the nosographic catalogs are regularly changed to include new diseases and to replace old diseases that have either disappeared or received new titles. Among these nosographic catalogs are the *International Classification of Diseases* (which is revised every ten years),[20] the *Systematized Nomenclature of Pathology,*[16] and the *Diagnostic and Statistical Manual of Mental Disorders* (now in a third edition).[146]

The second process of classification is an act of diagnosis. It is the clinimetric activity that occurs whenever a clinician reviews the existing nosographic catalog and chooses the appropriate diagnostic titles for a particular patient. For a patient with chest pain, the catalog may contain such diagnostic possibilities as pneumonia, esophageal stricture, fractured rib, and myocardial infarction. The clinician's clinimetric challenge is to decide which of the available diagnoses is most suitable.

For this task, the clinician uses diagnostic criteria that provide operating specifications for making a clinical decision about the existence of a particular disease. If the disease is defined morphologically, the clinimetric index—such as the WHO criteria for diagnosis of myocardial infarction[92]—will contain operating specifications for making a clinical diagnosis when the definitive morphologic evidence is not readily available. If the disease is not defined morphologically, the clinimetric index—as in the Jones diagnostic criteria for rheumatic fever—can serve both to define the disease and to provide specifications for its diagnosis.

2.3.1.2. *Ratings of Clinical Conditions*

A different type of clinimetric index serves to characterize a particular condition. If the condition has already been identified as a disease, such as myocardial infarction or rheumatic fever, the index may then add such descriptive adjectives as *acute, severe,* or *recurrent.* In many other instances, however, the condition refers to a functional status, rather than a disease, and the clinimetric index provides a rating for that status. Among such indexes are the Apgar score for the condition of a newborn baby, the Glasgow coma scale, and the New York Heart Association classification of cardiac disability.

2.3.1.3. *Therapeutic Agents*

Most of the therapeutic agents used in clinical practice are identified according to the standard nomenclature of pharmaceutical regimens or surgical operations, but other interventions may require description in clinimetric indexes. Such indexes might be needed, for example, to describe patterns of nutrition, physical activities, or types of biofeedback mechanisms. The term *bedside manner* is commonly used to refer to the particular therapeutic assistance provided by a clinician's style of communication, reassurance, and compassion. Other important therapeutic adjuncts that may require specific clinimetric identifications are social support systems and familial interrelationships.

2.3.2. INDEXES OF CHANGE

A patient's condition can be changed by the new occurrence of something, such as an acute myocardial infarction, that was not present before, or by the disappearance, such as a completely resolved pneumonia, of a previous event. In these types of straightforward appearance or disappearance, the subsequent status of the event can usually be identified with the same kind of status index that was previously used to note its initial presence or absence.

In some circumstances, however, the subsequent event may be a recurrence rather than a completely new appearance, or a remission rather than a total disappearance. Because different diagnostic criteria may be needed to identify recurrences, remissions, or other evolutions of a previous condition, the indexes used for describing the initial status of an event may be modified for use in describing outcomes or subsequent status.

In most considerations of change, however, the entity under observation is an adjective, describing the magnitude or some other graded attribute of a particular state, rather than its mere existence. We might want to know about alterations in blood pressure, pain, severity of illness, or degree of disability. This type of change, which usually involves a comparison of two (or more) states, can be cited in at least two different ways.

In the most common approach, the patient's subsequent condition is repeatedly cited with the same type of status index that was used to describe the previous condition. The "before" and "after" values of this index can then be directly compared, usually by subtraction, to indicate the change. Thus, if the patient's grip strength was **149 mm Hg** before treatment and is **133 mm Hg** afterward, the change can be expressed as a **fall of 16 mm Hg.** This type of change is cited dyadically, with a direct comparison of previous and subsequent values for a single status index. The expression of a dyadic change does not always require dimensional data. For example, if functional condition is **Grade IV** before treatment and **Grade III** afterward, the change could be cited as **improvement of one grade.**

When more than two values of a single status index are included in the total measurement, the "polyadic" index of change can be summarized with various statistical expressions, such as a mean or regression line for the individual values. Alternatively, the series of values can be given a categorical rating, such as **normal** or **abnormal** for the pattern of successive values in a glucose tolerance test.

In a different approach, a change can be cited "monadically," with a distinctive, separate transition index, which does not contain a specific citation for the previous values of an analogous status index. In a classic example of a dyadic approach to an index for change of pain, we might ask a patient to rate the severity of his pain on a scale of **1, 2, 3, 4, 5** before and after treatment. The two ratings would then be compared to determine the change. In a monadic approach, we might ask a treated patient to use a scale of **−2, −1, 0, +1, +2** or a scale of **better, same, worse** for answering the question, "How is your pain now compared with what it was before treatment?" Although the patient would recall his previous condition when answering this question, the response would be cited in a monadic value that does not require citation of a specific rating for either the pre- or post-treatment severity of pain.

In a monadic rating of change, the entities under appraisal can be two individual states, a series of states, or the total pattern of response. The rating for the change can be an evaluation such as **excellent** or **poor;** a comparative term such as **larger, worse, unchanged, improved,** or **deteriorating;** or a numerical ranking in a scale such as **−2, −1, 0, +1, +2.**

Special monadic indexes of change, called *transition indexes,* are often needed to distinguish differences that can occur while the patient remains in the same category of a status index. Thus, a patient who has become able to feed himself while still unable to ambulate may be listed as **incapacitated** in both the pre-treatment and post-treatment ratings of a status index of functional ability. A comparison of these two ratings would show no apparent change and the patient's improvement would not be discerned unless a special index were used to focus on transitions in functional ability.

2.3.3. PROGNOSTIC INDEXES

A prognostic index is used to predict an outcome, which is a future rather than current status. The prediction may be expressed quantitatively in an expression such as **30% five-year survival rate,** or in verbal terms, such as **good, impending,** or **hopeless.** Most prognostic indexes are status indexes that have been given an additional predictive role. For example, a *TNM Stage* is often used as a status index to rate the condition of patients with cancer, but the same index is also used for prognostic estimations. The estimate might be expressed as "the expected five-year survival rate is 30% for a patient who is in **TNM Stage III.**"

Although often mentioned and illustrated at various places in this book, prognostic indexes will not be extensively discussed. Indexes of status and change occur much more commonly in clinical work; and the evaluation of prognostic indexes would require a detailed appraisal of methods used for prediction itself, not just the structure of predictive indexes. An analytic evaluation of all the methods used for clinical prognostication would be worthwhile, but is well beyond the scope of a relatively short text.

2.3.4. CLINICAL GUIDELINES

A clinimetric index is used as a clinical guideline when it provides specific instructions for an action decision, such as ordering a diagnostic test, or choosing or discontinuing a particular treatment. A status index becomes a guideline when accompanied by an appropriate statement such as "surgery is contra-indicated for patients in TNM Stage III." After treatment is begun, a status index can become a guideline by identifying a subsequent clinical condition that mandates the cessation of therapy. Thus, a particular treatment may be stopped if, according to appropriate indexes, the patient either deteriorates or develops an adverse drug reaction. The role of the index in this situation is to demarcate the characteristics of the deterioration or adverse drug reaction that warrant the therapeutic decision.

Although instructions about what to do next can be appended to a conventional status index, many clinical-guideline indexes have been specially constructed as algorithms or flow-charts that indicate the actions to be taken in response to different clinical situations. The name *protocol* has sometimes been used when the guidelines are intended for nurse practitioners, physicians' assistants, or other nonphysicians. With certain special formats, guideline indexes have been used for medical audit procedures in evaluating clinical performance or competence in health care activities. Komaroff,[102,103] Greenfield,[72,73] and their colleagues have been particularly active in developing algorithm-protocol-guideline procedures.

The construction and evaluation of guideline indexes will also receive relatively little attention here. The guideline indexes are usually intended to offer directions for making "action" decisions, rather than to produce data used for scientific or statistical analysis. The instructions offered in a guideline must be clear enough to be understood by potential users, but the scientific quality of a guideline will depend on the decisions to which it leads, not on the guideline itself. For example, if the guideline indicates when to order a particular test for a patient with acute urinary symptoms, the decision must be justified by appropriate evidence showing the value of the ordered test. Regardless of how the guideline index is constructed—as an algorithm, decision table, or verbal text—the key scientific issue will be the justifying evidence rather than the format and contents of the index. Another topic beyond the scope of the discussion here is the type of authoritative recommendations, often called *guidelines,* that may be offered for such health care activities as organizing a cardiac catheterization laboratory or an intensive care unit. Guidelines of this type can be greatly helpful in administrative activities, but do not directly produce the types of index under discussion.

2.4. Architectural and Statistical Roles

Beyond the cited common clinical functions, every clinical index can be mathematically regarded as a *variable,* which provides data used in research and in statistical analysis of the results.

The research can be designed for diverse purposes and with diverse architectural arrangements.[54] The purposes can include a purely descriptive account of what is happening or a comparison planned for decisions about cause-effect relationships or the quality of processes. The cause-effect investigations can be concerned with etiology of disease, physiologic or pathophysiologic mechanisms, pharmacologic actions, or therapeutic interventions used for prophylactic, salutary, or remedial purposes. The quality of processes can be studied for chemical measurements, the efficacy of diagnostic marker tests, observer variability in subjective decisions, or audits of the plans made in a patient's management. The architectural arrangements used in the research can include a case series, a randomized experimental trial, an observational cohort study, a case-control study, a secular or ecologic association, or various other formats for assembling groups and comparing their data.

The data collected with these diverse architectural purposes and structures are usually summarized statistically and subjected to statistical analyses, which lead to the conclusions drawn in the research. The basic information used in these analyses is often cited in clinical indexes. The data provided by the indexes have become the fundamental sources of identification for the groups, conditions, spectrums, and associations that are expressed statistically as the final result of the investigative activities.

The six sections that follow contain further discussion of the various ways in which the basic data of clinimetric indexes are transformed into the statistical results of clinical research. The sections are in smaller type to indicate that they are optional reading—available for someone who wants to know the details but unnecessary for someone who wants to get on with it and stick to the essentials. Readers who prefer to avoid the extra details should proceed directly to Section 2.5.

2.4.1. DELINEATION OF A GROUP

A prime statistical role of diagnostic criteria and other status indexes is to demarcate the particular group of people (or other entities) under analysis. The index will show which people should or should not be counted when we determine N, the size of the group under study.

The specifications supplied by the index are usually called *admission criteria* for the investigated group; and the admission criteria usually contain subsets of criteria having three different functions. The *eligibility criteria* denote the relatively coarse qualifications that each person must fulfill to be considered as a candidate for admission. These qualifications, which are often cited with general diagnostic criteria, may then be refined with additional specifications for the inclusion or exclusion of eligible candidates.

Within the group of people who fulfill the general eligibility criteria, *inclusion criteria* are often used to delineate a subgroup of people who are the focus of a particular study. For example, among patients who satisfy the diagnostic criteria for acute myocardial infarction, the investigators may want to concentrate on only those patients who had stable angina pectoris before the infarction. The status index that defines "stable angina pectoris" will be the inclusion criterion that creates a diagnosis within a diagnosis, circumscribing the larger entity into a smaller focus of investigation.

A status index can also circumscribe the focus of the research by excluding a particular subgroup of otherwise eligible people. Thus, in studying patients with acute myocardial infarction and previously stable angina pectoris, the investigators may use *exclusion criteria* that define and eliminate people who are "too old," or who have had "antecedent congestive heart failure."

The circumscribing indexes used for inclusions or exclusions are really subsets of eligibility indexes, but they are cited here as separate entities because certain indexes are used (and can be evaluated) for only the circumscribing function.

2.4.2. FOCAL CONDITION FOR A GROUP

Although the admission criteria delineate the denominator as a group of people under study, most of the excitement in the research is provided by information that indicates the focal condition selected as a numerator. The focal condition can be cross-sectional, noted when the basic group is examined, or a longitudinal outcome phenomenon, noted after the members of the group are followed forward in time. For example, *antecedent myocardial infarction* or *baseline cholesterol value* might be noted as cross-sectional prevalent conditions in a group of people; and *subsequent myocardial infarction* and *reduction in cholesterol* might be observed as longitudinal incidence conditions when the group is followed forward in time.

Clinimetric indexes are regularly used to identify the antecedent, concurrent, or subsequent states that become the focal conditions examined as numerators in the research.

2.4.3. DISTRIBUTION OF A SPECTRUM

The information assembled for the focal condition of each member of a group shows the *spectrum* of data for that condition; and the distribution of the spectrum is regularly summarized with an appropriate statistical expression. For dimensional data, such as *age* or *weight,* the summary expressions may be a mean and standard deviation, or a median and inner-95-percentile range.[54] For a binary-data event, such as the concomitant (or future) presence or absence of a myocardial infarction, the summary expression might be a proportion showing a rate of occurrence for the event. If the spectrum contains a series of unranked categories for a nominal variable, such as race or religion, the summary expression would indicate the proportions (or relative frequency) or each category found in the spectrum. If the data contain ranked grades (such as *TNM Stage or rating for pain*), different data analysts may summarize the spectrum in different ways. Some analysts will cite the results only as proportions for each categorical grade. Other analysts will assign arbitrary numerical values to the categories—such as 0 = none, 1 = mild, 2 = moderate, 3 = severe—and the results will be summarized with means, standard deviations, or other expressions used for dimensional data.

Regardless of how they are formed, spectral summaries constantly serve as prime expressions of the results of research. The expressions can be used for purely descriptive purposes, or for comparisons intended to show the similarity or disparity of two contrasted groups.

2.4.3.1. *Denominator Resemblances*

The spectral distribution of two groups is commonly contrasted to show their *denominator,* or *baseline resemblance* in cogent factors other than the main focal event(s) under consideration in the research. The contrast may be done for such purposes as showing that two treated groups had similar severity of clinical illness before the treatments were imposed, or that the case and control groups in an etiologic case-control study were similar in age, gender, diagnostic surveillance, and all other cogent attributes except the antecedent exposure that was the main focal condition under investigation.

2.4.3.2. *Focal Disparities*

Although certain attributes are regularly examined for similarity, the most frequent reason for contrasting the spectrum of two groups is to show a focal disparity. The usual goal is to demonstrate a difference that is "statistically significant" for such focal conditions as the outcome events of compared treatments, or the antecedent exposures of case and control groups. Most of these contrasts are carried out by comparing the spectrum of a selected index in the two groups, and the results are usually expressed statistically with increments, ratios, or proportional increments.[54]

For example, the ratings of a clinimetric index of co-morbidity may be summarized and contrasted to show that two groups of diabetic patients, despite randomized assignment of therapy, had a significant difference in baseline severity of pre-existing disease before the compared treatments were initiated. Summary ratings of quality of life may be contrasted to show that outcomes after surgery were better than after medical therapy for coronary artery disease. Ratios derived from counts of an index of previous "exposure to occupational toxin" may be analyzed to imply that such exposure can lead to the deleterious outcome noted in the case group of a case-control study.

2.4.4. ASSOCIATIONS FOR TREND

Two or more variables (or groups) are commonly associated statistically to show the trend of their relationships. For example, data for two variables, *TNM Stage* and *severity of pain,* in a group of patients with cancer might be associated to examine the relationship between the spread of the cancer (TNM Stage) and its symptomatic effects.

The association can be simple, containing only two variables, or multivariate. In the latter instance, we might examine the relationship between severity of pain and a set of several variables, such as TNM stage, duration of illness, co-morbidity, and socioeconomic status. The association can be demonstrated directly with a graph or cross-tabulation, or estimated with a mathematical model, such as a line, plane, or multi-dimensional "surface." Clinimetric indexes can be used to identify any of the variables or groups that are analyzed in the simple or multivariate associations.

Beyond their role as variables examined in associations, clinical indexes may themselves be formed by an association process. Thus, a set of several variables may be mathematically aggregated in a multivariate association to form an index that is a single score, or a "factor" composed of a smaller set of weighted variables. The mathematical processes used to form such indexes are discussed further in Chapter 8.

The mathematical trend of a relationship is often arranged in the form of a cause-effect model, with a dependent variable having the role of effect and an independent variable (or variables) having the role of cause. This was the type of dependency relationship that was considered earlier when severity of pain was regarded as being possibly affected by a combination of TNM Stage, duration of illness, co-morbidity, and socioeconomic status. The main hazard of the cause-effect structure used in these mathematical models, as discussed elsewhere,[54] is that reality may not always coincide with the basic ideas of the model. The mathematical manifestations of causal dependency may arise only because of various biases or other defects in the architecture of the research.

2.4.5. STRATIFICATIONS

Stratifications are cross-tabulations of data, intended to display specific evidence for evaluating trends. As discussed later in Chapter 8, the statistical method of describing a trend is to cite a coefficient of correlation or regression. The coefficient provides an excellent summary of the relationship, but the actual data are not displayed. For example, the relationship between gender and survival can be expressed with a coefficient of association, but we would not see the actual evidence. A stratified cross-tabulation, presented in a 2 × 2 table that has **male** and **female** as categories of gender and **alive** and **dead** as categories of survival, would show the numbers that constitute the actual data for the four pertinent groups. The value of these direct displays of clinimetric evidence will also be discussed in Chapter 8.

In addition to making the evidence of an association easy to see and understand, stratifications are particularly helpful in the clinical interpretation of results for therapeutic and other agents that may have a cause-effect impact. Instead of examining the results for everyone who has received two compared treatments, we can perform a stratified comparison in which each of the treatments is compared within cogent clinical subgroups, which are called *strata*. Thus, we might compare the success rates of radiotherapy vs. chemotherapy not for all patients with a particular cancer, but for strata of patients in **Stage I, Stage II,** and **Stage III.** Since the strata are often formed from combinations of many variables, an important challenge in clinimetrics is to select and aggregate the particular variables that will form the best demarcation of strata for this or other comparative purposes.

2.4.6. CONCORDANCES

All of the associations just cited were intended to demonstrate trends in the relationship among *different* variables. In studies of observer variability and in other forms of process research, however, the statistical association may express agreement or concordance in different measurements of the *same* variable. For example, if severity of illness for each member of a group of patients is rated by one clinician whose ratings are compared with those made independently by a second clinician, the two sets of ratings would be analyzed for their agreement, not just for trend alone. The statistical indexes used to cite concordance[54] are often such calculations as percentage agreement, kappa coefficient, or intraclass correlation coefficient.

2.5. Framework of an Index

The classification just cited for architectural and statistical functions is important for determining how well an index does its assigned job. An index that is good for demarcating admission criteria may not be satisfactory for identifying outcome events. An index that is poor for contrasting spectrums may be excellent for making predictive correlations. An index that is excellent for showing stratified comparisons may not be good for testing observer variability.

In addition to checking the function of an index when we evaluate it, we also need to know the *framework* of the particular clinical setting in which the index is employed. The contents that make an index good may depend on whether the index is used for men or for women, for different age groups, or for special occupations or hospital locations. Aside from these demographic distinctions, the contents of a good index may depend on the particular nuances of the clinical situation. For example, the diagnostic criteria for acute myocardial infarction will differ if used to admit patients to a study of acute immediate treatment or to a study of long-term therapy begun after discharge from the hospital. The types of patients admitted to a study of chemotherapy for cancer will differ if the admission criteria require histologic, cytologic, or no microscopic evidence of the cancer.

For these reasons, the evaluation of a clinimetric index requires consideration of both the functional role of the index and the framework in which it is employed. These principles of evaluation can be borne in mind and saved for future usage as we turn, in the next few chapters, to the methods used in constructing clinimetric indexes.

Chapter 3

Basic Principles in the Structure of Clinimetric Indexes

In the customary forms of scientific mensuration, we first choose a particular attribute, such as age or serum cholesterol concentration, as the focus of attention. We then develop an appropriate method for measuring the magnitude of that attribute and expressing the results. When these decisions are converted into data, the attribute is called a *variable,* and the results are cited in a *scale* of available categories. The scale usually contains an array of successive dimensions, such as **..., 37, 38, 39, ... years of age** or **..., 265, 266, 267, ... mg/dl.** When the scales are applied to individual persons, the results are called *values.* Thus, someone might have the values of **39** for years of age and **167** for serum cholesterol concentration.

This same basic process takes place in clinimetric mensuration, but the process is much more complicated. Although the data produced by any method of measurement can be regarded as a variable, the name *index* is often reserved for variables that are formed as a mixture of two or more underlying variables, which are called the *components* of the index. Thus, the *Apgar Score*[5] is an index formed from five component variables, which refer to *heart rate, respiratory rate, color, muscle tone,* and *reflex response to nasal catheter.* Each of the component variables has its own rating scale, containing the three categories **0, 1,** and **2;** and the Apgar Score is formed as the sum of the five ratings.

The Apgar scoring process illustrates two of the main distinctions between clinimetric indexes and customary forms of laboratory measurement: the first distinction is the use of rating scales that contain arbitrary nondimensional categories, such as **0, 1, 2;** the second distinction is the formation of an index as a combination of ratings for multiple variables. The opportunity to use non-dimensional scales and multiple variables is what makes clinimetric indexes so versatile and important, but it also makes them complex. The complexity is particularly apparent when composite indexes are constructed as combinations of two or more component variables. Differences can occur in the scales of expression used for the component variables, in the ways the variables are combined, and in the scale used to express the output.

If only one variable is involved, the index has a simple construction. The single variable is chosen and expressed in a suitable scale. When several variables are included in a composite index, the sequence of construction is outlined in Figure 3.1. In the first step a series of candidate variables is examined, and certain variables are eliminated, leaving the component variables that will be included in the index. The scales for those component variables may have been selected beforehand; if not, their scales are demarcated at this step. In the next step, the component variables are combined. They may be joined directly to form the output scale, or they may first be combined into axes (or subscales). If axes are used, the output scale is then formed from combinations of the axes.

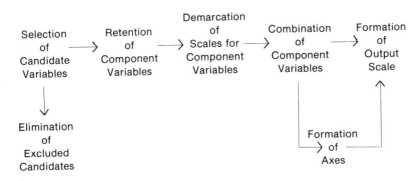

Figure 3.1. Sequence of Construction for a Composite Index

The complexities of this construction process will be discussed in three chapters. The rest of this chapter is concerned with the scales used for either a simple or a composite index and with the ways in which component variables are combined. Chapter 4 is devoted to the choice of component variables, and Chapter 5 to the organization of the output scale.

3.1. **Categories for Expressing Scales**

In providing the collection of categories available for expressing a particular class of data, a scale can refer to either a simple single variable or the output of a composite index, containing multiple input components. For example, heart rate is a single variable expressed in a dimensional scale of ..., **89, 90, 91,** ... beats per minute. When used as a component of the Apgar score, heart rate is converted into an ordinal scale having the categories **0, 1,** and **2.** The values of these categories, and analogous values from the four other component variables, are added to form the Apgar score's output scale, which is **0, 1, 2, ..., 10.**

This section contains a classification of different types of scales, regardless of whether the scales refer to a single variable or to the output of a composite variable.

3.1.1. DISTINCTIONS IN RANKING

Scales are usually classified according to the precision with which their categories can be ranked. At one extreme is a dimensional scale, whose categories can be measured and ranked with high precision. At the other extreme is a nominal scale, whose categories have no magnitudes and cannot be ranked. Between these extremes are three other scales, containing ordinal, quasi-dimensional, and binary categories. These five types of scale are discussed in the sections that follow.

3.1.1.1. *Nominal Scales*

The categories of a nominal scale have no overt order or ranking. For example, the scale for *religion* contains an unrankable set of categories such as **Buddhist, Christian, Jewish, Mohammedan,** and **Other.** Nominal scales are also formed by the collections of unranked categories used to express such variables as occupation, race, or ethnic background.

3.1.1.2. *Dimensional Scales*

In a ranked scale, the categories can be arranged according to their relative magnitudes, which are either dimensional or ordinal. In a dimensional scale, any two adjacent categories have magnitudes that are separated by a measurably equal interval. The previously cited expressions for age in years and serum cholesterol concentration were examples of dimensional scales. Because of the equi-interval attribute, dimensional scales are sometimes called *interval* scales, but the word *dimensional* seems preferable to avoid the connotation of *interval* as an expression of time.

A dimensional scale can have either integer categories, such as **0, 1, 2, 3,...** for number of children, or continuous values, which can be measured, when appropriate, with such increasing degrees of precision as **135, 135.2, 135.17,** or **135.168** for weight in pounds.

3.1.1.3. *Ordinal Scales*

In an ordinal scale, the adjacent categories can be ranked in a monotonically ascending or descending sequence of magnitude, but the categories are assigned arbitrarily and the intervals between them cannot be actually measured. An example of an ordinal scale is **mild, moderate,** and **severe** for degree of dyspnea, or **Class I, II, III,** or **IV** for the New York Heart Association Functional Classification.[24] Most of the ordinal scales used in clinical work contain a set of arbitrary grades, such as the two examples just cited, or the categories of **0, 1+, 2+, 3+,** and **4+** that are commonly used in clinical discourse. A different type of ordinal scale contains rankings rather than grades. A ranking occurs when members of a class are given successive numbers, such as **1, 2, 3, 4, 5,..., 67, 68,...,** according to their rank in class standing, or when medical students list their order of preferred choice of hospitals in the resident-matching plan.

3.1.1.4. *Quasi-Dimensional Scales*

When the numerical grades of several ordinal scales are combined, the output scale may seem to have dimensional characteristics. For example, when the five components of the Apgar score—each expressed in an ordinal scale of **0, 1,** or **2**—are added, the output scale has an apparently dimensional range from **0** to **10.** A similar process occurs when arbitrary ratings are assigned and then added as point scores for answers to the individual questions in a certifying test or examination of clinical competence. The output scale, created as the sum of these ordinal ratings, will be a score having such apparently dimensional values as **37, 98,** or **426.** The term *quasi-dimensional* can be used for these composite ordinal scales.

Another type of quasi-dimensional ordinal scale is called a *visual analog* scale. It consists of a line on which the observer is asked to mark the degree of a subjective sensation, such as pain or satisfaction. The line contains a measured length, often 100 mm, with the extreme ratings noted at either end. Thus, an index for satisfaction with health care might be constructed by asking a patient to mark a point on the following line:

├──┤

Totally
Dissatisfied

Totally
Satisfied

If the patient marks a point that is two thirds of the distance between **totally dissatisfied,** at one end of the line, and **totally satisfied,** at the other end, the index for satisfaction with health care might be scored as **0.67.** Because criteria for measurably equal intervals are not established between adjacent categories of the numerical ratings, visual analog scales are often regarded as ordinal or quasi-dimensional rather than dimensional.

3.1.1.5. *Binary Scales*

A binary or dichotomous scale contains only two categories, such as **alive** or **dead, male** or **female.** The scales are commonly used to express the presence or absence of a particular entity, and the citation is often **yes** or **no** (or **present** or **absent**) for such attributes as diagnosis of rheumatic fever, existence of chest pain, or occurrence of antecedent myocardial infarction. Because binary scales usually refer to an entity's existence, they are sometimes called *existential scales.* When *gender* is cited in the two binary categories of **male** or **female,** the scale seems nominal, but it becomes more obviously existential if converted to expression as **yes** or **no** for *presence of male gender.*

Most existential binary scales can be regarded as a subset of ordinal scales. The categories of **no** and **yes** (or **absent** or **present**) are often assigned coding values of **0** or **1,** which can be statistically analyzed as ordinal (or quasi-dimensional) data. The ordinal characteristic of an existential scale becomes more evident when the gradations of existence are expanded into an array such as **definitely present, probably present, uncertain whether present or absent, probably absent,** and **definitely absent.**

In ascending order of precision in ranking, the five main types of scales (and the indexes or data associated with them) can be classified as *nominal, binary, ordinal, quasi-dimensional,* and *dimensional.*

3.1.2. ADDITIONAL FORMATS AND NOMENCLATURE

The types of scales just cited are also used, particularly by psychosocial scientists, with somewhat different formats and nomenclature. The scales are usually arranged in a manner that allows them to be self-administered, with the respondent making a mark that indicates the selected choice.

A simple ordinal scale, having a set of individually identified ranked categories, is usually called a *specific category scale.* In the typical arrangement, a diabetic patient might be asked to respond with one of the following choices to the statement, "Testing my urine is..."

No trouble	*Some trouble,*	*A good bit,*	*A lot of*
at all	*but not much*	*but not a lot*	*trouble*

The selected categories can refer to rated grades (such as those just cited), frequencies (such as **always, usually, sometimes,** etc.), or degrees of agreement (such as **strongly agree, agree, uncertain,** etc.).

The term *differential scale* is used for a ranked ordinal scale having identified labels for its extreme categories but not for its intermediate categories. One main format for differential scales, discussed previously as a *visual analog scale,* contains a linear continuum of points that can be marked to provide quasi-dimensional values. The line can be placed vertically rather than horizontally, or it can take the form of an arc rather than a straight line. When interval descriptive labels are inserted (but not specifically marked) between the extreme boundaries of the line, the format is called a *graphic rating scale.* Thus, a standard visual analog scale would be displayed as:

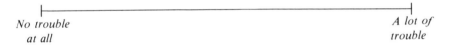

No trouble   *A lot of*
  at all   *trouble*

A graphic rating scale would be shown as:

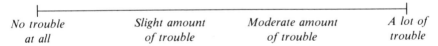

No trouble	*Slight amount*	*Moderate amount*	*A lot of*
at all	*of trouble*	*of trouble*	*trouble*

After comparing the utility of different formats and scales for measuring pain, *Sriwatanakul et al.*[148] concluded that visual analog scales may be more sensitive than conventional scales containing descriptive categories; that horizontal graphic lines were more desirable than vertical; and that the best scale (in their study) was a horizontal straight line with marked but unidentified intervals, as shown below:

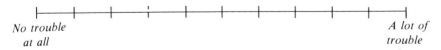

No trouble   *A lot of*
  at all   *trouble*

A second format for differential scales is called a *semantic differential scale.* It resembles an unlabeled, interval-marked visual analog scale. The respondent is asked, however, to choose a *category* among a series of demarcated grades rather than a *point* in a dimensional continuum. In this type of scale, the diabetic patient's response would be solicited as:

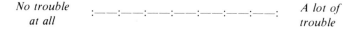

The semantic differential psychosocial scales usually contain seven categories because of the frequent belief[14,124] that seven graded categories are an optimum number in an ordinal scale.

3.1.3. NATURAL VS. ARBITRARY EXPRESSIONS

Before a scale is used, the original observation may have been described in whatever manner seemed appropriate or natural. This type of description is regularly encountered when archival information—such as the material contained in a patient's medical record—is being excerpted for analysis. During the excerption process, the original information is converted into variables and scales. Alternatively, if data are being solicited directly and if an appropriate scaling system does not exist for certain types of information, the observer may be asked to express things in a natural descriptive manner by filling in a blank.

The natural description may or may not be cited in the arbitrary categories of a scale. For example, most observers would record a person's age in years naturally as ..., **37, 38, 39,**... rather than citing such arbitrary categories as **young, middle,** or **old.** Similarly, a radiologist asked to express configuration of heart on a chest roentgenogram might prefer to make a natural brief description rather than to choose between the two arbitrary categories of **normal** and **abnormal.**

In both of these two instances, a distinctive choice existed, because relatively standard methods can be used to describe *age* and *configuration of heart* in either natural or arbitrary expressions. We could readily allow the observer to use a natural expression because we could easily transform it into an arbitrary scale. In fact, for entities such as age, the natural expression is a preferred mechanism for recording the original data.

In many other instances, however, a natural scale of expression does not exist. Whatever information is acquired as the raw data is recorded on an arbitrary scale. For example, because a natural scale does not exist for citing raw observational data about *briskness of neurologic reflexes,* clinicians regularly use such arbitrary ratings as **0, 1+,** or **2+.**

3.2. **Demarcation of Categories**

When we use an ordinary ruler to measure distance in cm, the available dimensional categories are clearly demarcated on the instrument, which shows the dimensional value directly. Analogously, the user of a nondimensional scale—such as **mild, moderate, severe**—needs feedback from the instrument to indicate how to choose the categories. This type of feedback is usually provided by a set of instructions or operational criteria that define and demarcate the categories. The demarcation will describe the particular attributes that distinguish **mild** from **moderate** from **severe** or the characteristics that might allow *existence of chest pain* to be rated as **yes** or **no.**

3.2.1. ABSENCE OF STIPULATIONS

Although instructions of this type are needed both for conventional forms of laboratory measurement and for clinimetric indexes, many clinical ratings are expressed in scales for which the categories are not demarcated. The user of the index is shown a list of available categories or the line of a visual analog scale, and is invited to choose a category or a location on the scale, but no specifications are cited to demarcate the categories. For example, the Killip Index of myocardial dysfunction, shown in Table 2.3, mentions venous hypertension, oliguria, and cyanosis, but does not cite criteria for identifying those entities. The Jones Diagnostic Criteria for rheumatic fever, shown in Table 2.4, do not contain thorough criteria for identifying such component entities as arthritis, carditis, chorea, and fever.

The absence of such stipulations, although at first suggestive of scientific delinquency, can often be reasonably justified after further reflection on reasons for the omissions. Wanting to have an index accepted and used for its important functional role, the developer of the clinical index may prefer to keep it relatively simple and non-controversial. The additional details needed to stipulate criteria for such entities as oliguria or carditis may be so extensive that potential clinical users of the index may find it too laborious, pedantic, unattractive, or repugnant. Furthermore, since an entity such as oliguria can be identified in diverse ways with different numerical boundaries for different clinical circumstances, the developer of the index may be reluctant to establish boundaries for all the circumstances, and may fear that whatever boundaries are chosen may evoke controversy. Accordingly, the developer may prefer to let the component entities be identified by the user's clinical judgment, which can be flexibly adapted for each circumstance, and which will make the index acceptable to that user.

For routine clinical application of an index, this approach may be quite satisfactory. If one clinician tells another that a patient is "4+ sick" or "in shock," the clinical condition is reasonably well appreciated by both clinicians, even though each may have different criteria for exact use of those terms. On the other hand, when the information is used in a research setting, the investigators may want to improve the reproducibility of the results by developing better stipulations for the component elements. Thus, a group of investigators, studying the subsequent clinical course of patients with rheumatic fever, augmented the basic structure of the Jones Diagnostic Criteria[3] by establishing additional criteria to stipulate the identification of carditis[37] and recurrent carditis.[39]

When clinimetric indexes are used in research, a prime scientific challenge will often be the development of additional criteria for stipulating the basic components. If the index is used in a setting where the investigators are prepared to devote the necessary attention and effort, the extra details required for reproducible stipulations can be as extensive as needed. If the index is to be disseminated beyond the research setting into ordinary clinical practice, however, the details may need to be shortened. The challenge would be to add enough details to improve the basic stipulations without making the stipulations so rigid or lengthy that the index becomes too difficult or too unappealing for ordinary usage.

3.2.2. SPECIFICATION OF COMPONENTS

When the *wind-chill factor* or *temperature-humidity index* is calculated as a composite score, each of the components is clearly specified. Similarly, each of the five components of the *Apgar Score* is stipulated and given an individual rating before the five values are added to form the output score.

In certain global clinimetric indexes, however, the component variables as well as the categorical demarcations may be left unidentified. For example, when a patient's *improvement* is rated on a global scale of **worse, same, somewhat better, much better,** we do not know how the categories were demarcated, but we also do not know what particular attributes were component variables when the global rating was chosen. Did the improvement refer to pain, dyspnea, appetite, functional capacity, mixtures of these features, or some other characteristics?

As discussed later in Chapter 7, the absence of specified components and demarcations can be both a major virtue and a major flaw of global scales. The virtue is that the scale produces a direct, simple, sensible rating for a complex phenomenon, such as *improvement*. The flaw is that the rating lacks the specifications that would allow different people to use it in a reproducible manner.

Global scales are constantly used in clinical activities to produce such expressions as **4+ sick, substantially better, excellent response,** or **very distressed.** Although a global scale is characterized by the absence of demarcated output categories, certain global scales are doubly global in that they also lack specifications for the component variables. The latter situation may not arise when global scales are used for single variables, such as shortness of breath or other discomforts that seem clearly identified. Thus, the component variables are reasonably well specified if a global scale of **0, 1+, 2+, 3+, 4+** is used to rate severity of dyspnea, but not if the same scale is used for severity of illness. When specifications are provided to identify each component variable and to demarcate the individual ratings within each variable, the output categories are created with *explicit criteria.* In global or other scales that lack suitable specifications, the output is achieved with *implicit criteria.*

3.3. Stipulation of Stimulus in Stimulus-Response Indexes

In many clinical indexes, the observed results occur spontaneously as a patient reacts to the customary events of daily life and the extra burdens imposed by illness. In many other indexes, however, the patient responds to a specific individual stimulus. The stimulus can often occur as an ordinary event in daily living, such as working at a job or walking up a flight of stairs, but sometimes the stimulus is deliberately imposed as part of the clinimetric activities. For example, a glucose tolerance test depends on the response of a patient's blood glucose to the stimulus of an ingested or injected load of glucose. Other stimulus-response indexes are produced when a patient walks a treadmill in an exercise tolerance test, breathes through a special apparatus in a pulmonary function test, or describes the images presented in a Rorschach test.

In such circumstances, the complete stipulation of the index requires that the stimulus as well as the observed responses be fully specified. Unless such specifications are offered, the stimulus cannot be adequately replicated, standardized, or evaluated for its contributions to the response. If the index produces inconsistent or unsuitable results, the absence of appropriate specifications for the stimulus may leave us unable to determine whether the problem arises from difficulties in selecting and replicating the stimulus, or from inadequacies in observing and rating the response.

An additional problem in stimulus-response indexes, however, occurs when the stimulus involves a delineated task—such as walking a marked distance as quickly as possible, or breathing deeply and rapidly—that requires cooperative effort by the patient. In such indexes, the response is usually rated according to the magnitude of the patient's performance, but adequate attention is seldom given to the patient's cooperative effort. This problem is so substantial and pervasive that it will receive separate attention, together with other clinimetric issues involving patients' active collaboration, in Chapter 6.

3.4. Combination of Components

One of the most distinctive features of clinimetric indexes is the combination of multiple component variables into a single output expression. In most forms of laboratory measurement, each variable is cited separately as an individual item of data, and each variable is used separately in subsequent analyses and calculations. In certain expressions, two or more variables may be mathematically combined to form a ratio, such as the Quetelet index or the albumin-globulin ratio; to calculate an increment, such as the anion gap; or to arrive at other mathematical products; but each variable is usually separately identified and specified in the calculations.

In many clinimetric indexes, however, the goal is to combine a large number of variables into a single output expression that will offer a rating for a complex clinical condition, such as a patient's state of health. Because so many variables are included, their individual identity is often deliberately omitted or inadvertently obscured in the output expression of the index. These multi-component indexes have always been used in an informal or global manner to answer such traditional medical questions as "How are you?", but a more formal arrangement has been needed for the quantitative assessments performed in modern medicine. The formal constructions have become particularly necessary for describing important human and clinical phenomena that cannot be discerned from the customary hard data provided by technologic measurements. Among such phenomena are severity of clinical illness, functional capacity, ability to conduct activities of daily living, and quality of life.

The choice and arrangement of variables in multi-component indexes is a prime clinimetric challenge that will be discussed in many locations of this book. The specific issues involved in formulating health status indexes, however, are too extensive for detailed attention here. Readers who want more information about health status indexes can find it in many other publications, which also contain listings of additional references.[8,29,71,95,98,122,138,147,153]

In the rest of this section, the emphasis is on the mechanisms used to construct a multi-component index. When contributions from more than one component variable are included, the output scale can be formed in many different arrangements. In one, the component ratings are preserved and cited individually, in tandem, to form what is often called a *profile*. In a more common combination, the component parts are aggregated or fused to create a new single expression. The aggregated expression is either an arithmetical score or a category, formed as a Boolean cluster of components; and the aggregates can be joined either as a nonspecific summation or as a specified hierarchy. The mechanisms of forming and arranging these combinations are discussed in the subsections that follow.

3.4.1. TANDEM PROFILES

A tandem profile contains a series of component variables that are cited together in a combination, but listed separately in tandem, without being fused into a distinctive new expression for the output scale. For example, the expression **T2N1M0** is a tandem profile for *TNM index,*[4] which denotes in this instance that the patient is in category **2** for tumor, category **1** for nodes, and category **0** for metastases. In a proposed index for severity of renal disease,[21] the final expression is a tandem profile identifying the individual state of three separate components—severity of signs and symptoms, severity of renal functional impairment, and level of performance of physical activity. The *Sickness Impact Profile,*[8] as shown by its name, is an index that contains a profile citation of twelve component variables, called subscales. They appear sequentially in the index as subscales concerned with sleep and rest, eating, work, home management, recreation and pastimes, ambulation, mobility, body care and movement, social interaction, alertness behavior, emotional behavior, and communication.

Since the individual components are each preserved without fusion into a composite output scale, tandem profile identifications have the advantage of not losing information. On the other hand, because the many possible varieties of expression cannot be easily ranked and are generally too large to permit useful analyses and comparisons, profile identifications are seldom employed except as pure descriptions. For analytic purposes, they are often converted into other forms of expression. For example, such TNM profiles as **T1N0M0, T2N0M0,** and **T1N1M0** cannot be used effectively to evaluate prognosis or treatment of cancer. The TNM profiles are therefore clustered into an ordinal set of TNM stages, such as **I, II,** and **III.**

3.4.2. AGGREGATIONS

The aggregation of different components into a single output scale is a distinctive clinimetric tactic that allows a complex phenomenon to be cited with one rating for the entire phenomenon. Such single ratings have readily been achieved and frequently used for clinical communication in global expressions—such as **2+ sick, poor condition,** or **moderately incapacitated**—for which the individual observational components and demarcational criteria are not specified. The main advantage of an aggregated index is that its single overall rating is achieved with deliberate specifications and demarcations for the components. The main disadvantage is that certain key distinctions in the component variables may be omitted, lost, or obscured in the multi-dimensional composite expression that emerges from the aggregation process.

3.4.2.1.   *Arithmetical Scores*

In an aggregated arithmetical score, the component variables are given numerical ratings and the ratings are joined mathematically. The most common mathematical procedure is an addition, as illustrated by the Apgar score, in which the values for the five component variables are summed to form the aggregate score. The component values need not always be added, however. The Quetelet Index of obesity is formed as a quotient when weight is divided by the squared value of height.[100]

In certain additive scores, the value of each component variable is multiplied by a coefficient, called a *weight* or *weighting factor,* before the addition takes place. This type of weighting commonly occurs when the elements are joined according to a specific mathematical process, such as multiple linear regression. For example, the *Norris Coronary Prognostic Index*[126] is created by the mathematical formula $3.9x_1 + 2.8x_2 + 10x_3 + 1.5x_4 + 3.3x_5 + 0.4x_6$. In this formula the individual x_i values are ratings for component variables identified as x_1 = age, x_2 = position of infarct, x_3 = admission systolic blood pressure, x_4 = heart size, x_5 = lung fields, and x_6 = previous ischemia.

3.4.2.2.   *Boolean Clusters*

In an aggregated Boolean cluster, the component variables are cited in categorical elements rather than in purely numerical values, and the output scale is formed when these elements are combined into clustered groups. Each output cluster in the scale is a separate category that is formed logically by the various unions and intersections of Boolean algebra. The categories may then be labeled with numerical, alphabetical, or verbal citations.

For example, the output scale of *TNM Stage* is a set of categories usually cited as **I, II,** and **III.** Each of these output categories is a Boolean cluster formed according to the presence or absence of various features of a cancer's topographic dissemination.[4] The categorical elements in these clusters might be demarcated as follows for the three stages of the output scale:

Stage I: Localized cancer *and* no evidence of regional spread *and* no evidence of distant metastasis

Stage II: Regional spread of cancer *and* no evidence of distant metastasis

Stage III: Any evidence of distant metastasis

For ease of remembrance, arbitrary numerical ratings are sometimes assigned to the individual component categories; and the result is expressed as a *scored cluster.* For example, suppose a rating of **1** is given for evidence of primary cancer, **2** for evidence of regional spread, and **4** for evidence of distant metastases. When these individual ratings are added together, a patient with a score of **1** would be in **Stage I.** Patients with scores of **2** or **3** would be in **Stage II.** Patients with scores of **4, 5, 6,** or **7** would be in **Stage III.**

Another composite scale formed with Boolean clusters is the Killip index for severity of myocardial derangement.[101] The output scale contains four ordinal categories: **no heart failure, heart failure, severe heart failure,** and **cardiogenic shock.** The categories are formed as various Boolean unions and intersections of component elements that include the following: rales, S_3 gallop, venous hypertension, hypotension, pulmonary edema, oliguria, cyanosis, and diaphoresis. The arrangement was shown earlier in Table 2.3.

Although every Boolean cluster forms a category, not all categorical scales are derived from clusters. For example, the dimensional values of serum cholesterol can be demarcated to form an ordinal scale expressed as **low, normal,** and **high.** The arithmetical values of an *Apgar Score* could be partitioned to form a scale such as **poor, fair, good,** and **excellent.** When statistical data are shown in the form of relative-frequency histograms or other graphical displays, dimensional values for a variable such as *age in years* are often grouped into ordinal categories such as **<20, 20–34, 35–49, 50–64, 65–79,** and **>79.**

3.4.3. SUMMATED VS. HIERARCHICAL AGGREGATES

When output scores or clusters are aggregated by direct fusion of the constituent components, the results can be arranged in a summated or hierarchical manner. In a summation, the component ratings are directly added (or joined in some other mathematical manner). Consequently, the same output scores can be achieved from the combination of several different component ratings. For example, an Apgar score of **5** can be attained if the component variables have ratings of **2+2+1+0+0,** or **0+0+2+2+1,** or **1+1+1+1+1,** or a variety of other patterns. If some of these patterns are more clinically important than others, the distinction cannot be discerned from the summated score of **5.** Similarly, when the Jones Criteria[3] form summated categorical clusters denoted as **yes** or **no** for the diagnosis of rheumatic fever, the positive rating does not indicate whether the patient has arthritis alone, carditis alone, or various mixtures of these (or other) categorical elements.

By contrast, a hierarchical arrangement contains a specific principle of ranking that identifies various categories as being more important than others. A patient is assigned to a higher (or lower) category of the output scale only if these cogent hierarchical distinctions are fulfilled. For example, in the TNM Staging system for cancer, a patient is first checked for distant metastatic lesions. If they are present, the patient is placed in **Stage III.** If distant metastases are absent, the patient is next checked for evidence of regional spread. If it is present, the assignment is **Stage II.** In the absence of either metastatic or regional spread, the patient is placed in **Stage I.** With this arrangement, we do not know whether a patient in **Stage III** does or does not have evidence of primary manifestations or regional spread—but we do know that the patient has distant metastases. An analogous type of hierarchical structure occurs in the Killip index, shown earlier in Table 2.3. If a patient is in Killip Class D, we do not know what other type of evidence is present for different degrees of congestive heart failure, but we know that the patient has cardiogenic shock.

Hierarchical arrangements can be achieved with special organization of either clustered or scored indexes. An example of the special scoring process was shown in Section 3.4.2.2 when numerical ratings of **1, 2,** and **4** were used respectively for primary, regional, and distant metastatic manifestations of a cancer. Because the scoring system is based on powers of 2—2^0, 2^1, and 2^2—anyone with a score of **4** or higher will be known to have distant metastases, and anyone with a score of **2** or **3** will be known to have regional spread. An example of the clustered arrangement for this same principle is shown in the Venn diagrams of Figure 3.2. The left-hand diagram shows the intersection of primary, regional, and distant manifestations to form seven possible categories. The right-hand diagram shows how these seven categories are demarcated to form three hierarchical stages.

Because of the more effective immediate communication, hierarchical arrangements are usually preferable to summations. The hierarchies are often more difficult to arrange, however, because they require complex decisions about importance, particularly when the index contains the multi-dimensionality of many component variables. In the case of the cited example for cancer staging, the hierarchy was easy to establish because it was based on

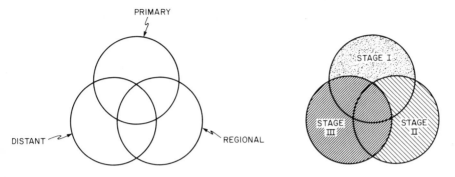

Figure 3.2. Boolean combination (on left) of three types of manifestations of a cancer. Demarcation (on right) of three hierarchical stages.

essentially a single variable, the extensiveness of the cancer's spread. In the case of the Killip index, the hierarchy depended on essentially two pathophysiologic variables—the magnitude of pump failure and the magnitude of hypoperfusion.

When more than two cogent variables are included in the index, a simple hierarchical arrangement may be more difficult to achieve. Thus, if cancer staging included such clinical variables as severity of symptoms, severity of co-morbidity, clinical rate of growth, and general functional capacity as well as the customary morphologic evidence of spread, a simple, logical hierarchy would be almost impossible to create. Patients could readily be classified at the extreme ends of the hierarchy, according to those with the best or worst ratings in each of the five variables. An intermediate set of hierarchical rankings, however, would not be easy to create or to recognize for patients with diverse combinations of good, bad, or in-between attributes.

Consequently, if an index contains only one or a few major variables, the decisions about importance are easy to make, and a hierarchical index is relatively easy to construct. If the index contains many variables and if the decisions are difficult, uncertain, or controversial, the summation process may be both easier and ultimately more effective than the construction of a disputed hierarchy. The hierarchical and summation procedures are discussed further in Chapter 9.

3.5. Formation of Axes

Before an output scale is formed, the component variables may first be aggregated into composite variables that are called *axes,* and the output scale is developed as a combination of the results in the scale for each axis. In certain indexes, these axes may be identified separately and called *subscales*. In a tandem profile, the output results are expressed as the rating for each of the subscales, but in other indexes, the subscales are aggregated into a single output expression.

For example, in the Jones diagnostic criteria,[3] evidence of such clinical features as arthritis, carditis, or chorea is collected into a *major* axis. Other types of evidence, such as certain abnormal laboratory tests, are collected in a *minor* axis. To give a positive result, the output scale requires evidence of two members in the major axis, or one member in the major axis *and* two members in the minor.

The WHO Diagnostic Criteria for myocardial infarction[92] depend on three major axes, which contain data about the patient's clinical history, electrocardiographic findings, and laboratory tests. Each of these axes contains a combination of the values for individual variables, such as characteristics of chest pain in the history, an account of Q waves and ST-T segments in the electrocardiogram, and results of creatine phosphokinase or other laboratory tests. Each axis is denoted as positive or negative according to certain criteria, and a positive result in the output scale requires certain combinations of positive results in the three axes.

An axis is formed whenever several individual variables are aggregated into a combination that then becomes a direct component of the output scale. For example, the M component of the TNM staging system for breast cancer is an axis labeled *evidence of distant metastases.* This axis contains a series of individual variables, each marked as **present** or **absent** according to evidence of metastasis to **brain, bone, liver, abdominal nodes,** etc. The axis is rated as **positive** if any one of the component variables is **present.**

For purposes of construction and evaluation, each axis can be regarded as an intermediate output scale. The axes are preserved as the subscales seen in a profile index; and the axes are fused to form the final output scale of an aggregated index. Because of these characteristics, the construction of an axis involves the same types of decisions previously discussed for aggregating variables to form a scale. The aggregate contained in the axis may be a score or a cluster, arranged in a summated or hierarchical fashion.

The frequent use of axes in clinimetric indexes increases the complexity of their structure and adds to the difficulties of providing satisfactory specifications for an index. The specifications will have to include the identity of each component variable, the demarcated rating scheme for the scale of that variable, the method of aggregating component variables into axes, the rating scheme for each axis, and the method of combining the axis ratings into the output scale.

3.6. **Transformation of Component Scales**

Before entering the primary component variables into a composite index, the investigator may sometimes alter their original scales. The conversions may downgrade a dimensional variable, upgrade a nominal variable into ordinal or dichotomous categories, or assign weighted ratings to an ordinal or dimensional variable. Other transformations may be imposed in accordance with certain scientific or statistical fashions.

3.6.1. DOWNGRADING OF DIMENSIONAL DATA

Dimensional data may be downgraded for several reasons. The goals may be to eliminate fine distinctions that are not cogent, to allow easy recall of the subsequent results, or to create categories similar to those used for other component variables in the aggregate index. The Apgar Score exemplifies all three of these goals when the dimensional values of heart rate are converted into the ordinal grades of **0** for *no heart beat evident,* **1** for *heart rate evident but below 100,* and **2** for *heart rate at least 100 per minute.* The **0, 1,** and **2** ordinal ratings are easy to remember; they contain the same scale as the other grades used in the Apgar score's non-dimensional component variables (such as color or tone); and the boundary of 100 acts as a useful demarcation between worrisome and nontroubling heart rates.

A more complicated example of ordinal downgrading for dimensional data appears in the Norris Prognostic Index[126] of coronary disease. The conversion transforms age in years from a dimensional to an ordinal scale in the following manner: $<50 = \mathbf{0.2}$; $50-59 = \mathbf{0.4}$; $60-69 = \mathbf{0.6}$; $70-79 = \mathbf{0.8}$; and $80-89 = \mathbf{1.0}$. An analogous transformation, producing the arbitrary ordinal categories of **0, 0.1, 0.2,..., 0.7,** and **1** is used in the Norris index to convert systolic blood pressure from dimensional values into grades.

In a disease activity score for Crohn's disease,[157] dimensional data are converted into a binary scale. Thus, *erythrocyte sedimentation rate* is graded as **1** (elevated) if the dimensional value is >20 mm, and as **0** (not elevated) for values <20 mm.

3.6.2. ORDINALIZATION OF NOMINAL DATA

Although nominal data have no inherent ranks, a grade can sometimes be assigned if suitable distinctions have been demonstrated. In this way, a nominal variable, such as *position of infarct,* becomes ordinalized in the Norris Prognostic Index when the following ordinal grades are assigned to the location of the myocardial infarction: *anterior transmural* = **1.0;** *posterior* *transmural* = **0.7**; *anterior subendocardial* = **0.3**; and *posterior subendo-cardial* = **0.3.**

3.6.3. DICHOTOMIZATION OF NOMINAL DATA

A different type of transformation is often used to prevent confusion when nominal data are given arbitrary code numbers—somewhat like Social Security or telephone numbers—that are used for storing information in a computer format. Thus, to store data for a nominal variable such as type of therapy, the coding digits of **1** might be used for Treatment A, **2** for Treatment B, **3** for Treatment C, and **4** for Treatment D. If these code numbers received a direct statistical analysis, however, the four digits might be regarded as ordinal or dimensional rankings rather than as nominal coding identifications.

To avoid this problem, the four nominal categories of the single variable, *type of treatment,* can be converted into four contrived binary variables that are sometimes called *dummy variables.* Each of these contrived binary variables would be scaled as **yes** or **no,** and the four variables would refer, successively, to the binary presence or absence of *Treatment A, Treatment B, Treatment C,* or *Treatment D.* If the four treatments are mutually exclusive (i.e., a patient can receive only one of them), a separate binary variable would not be needed for *Treatment D,* since it would be identified by a **no** value for each of the three other treatments.

3.6.4 WEIGHTED RATINGS

When the numerical rating of a variable is added (or used in some other mathematical manner), the impact of the variable in the total score can be altered by weighting its ratings. The weighting can be accomplished by changing the values of the individual ratings, or by multiplying them with a coefficient. For example, suppose an output score is obtained as the sum of ratings for three variables, expressed as $x_1 + x_2 + x_3$. If each of the three variables is cited in a scale of **0, 1,** and **2** (as in the Apgar score), the three variables have equal weights in their rating scales. If we think variable x_3 is twice as important as the other two variables, however, we can either change the scale of x_3 to **0, 2,** and **4,** or we can let the original scales remain intact while changing the aggregate score to $x_1 + x_2 + 2x_3$. In the latter instance, the 2 is a weighting coefficient, or weight for variable x_3.

An illustration of this process occurs in the Peel coronary prognostic index,[130] where the ordinal variables of different components have different rating scales. Thus, the scale for *heart failure* is **0, 1, 4,** whereas *shock* is rated as **0, 1, 5,** or **7.** Another illustration of this process was shown earlier (Section 3.4.2.1) when weighted ratings of **1.0, 0.7,** or **0.3** were assigned to categories for *location of myocardial infarction* in the Norris coronary prognostic index.

Decisions about the magnitude of the weights can be made with purely judgmental strategies or with the aid of some of the mathematical models discussed in chapter 8.

3.6.5. HIERARCHICAL WEIGHTS

In the weighted ratings just discussed, the weights were chosen according to the relative importance of each variable and of the categories within that variable. A substantially different basic approach may be needed when a hierarchical arrangement is desired for weights that are added together from several different variables. The patterns of the weighting may rely on powers of 2—as illustrated earlier in Section 3.4.3—or on other appropriate arrangements. Because of the complexity, a satisfactory set of weightings will usually be difficult to achieve when multiple variables are combined to form a hierarchy rather than a summation.

3.6.6. FASHIONS IN TRANSFORMATION

Certain other basic scales are transformed not for the clinimetric reasons cited in the four preceding sections but for preferences in scientific or statistical fashions. The scientific preferences may lead to the conversion of measured units from **lb.** to **kg., miles** to **km.,** and **°F** to **°C,** or vice versa. Statistical preferences for getting a Gaussian distribution in the spectrum of data may transform the basic measurements into logarithms, square roots, or arc sines of the original values. A transformed measurement, rather than the original scale, may sometimes become the standard unit of expression for the phenomenon. Thus, the conversion of hydrogen ion concentration to a negative logarithm has made the data easy to work with; and the pH value, which is the transformed negative logarithm of the measured concentration, has now become the standard mode of expression.

Since these fashions in transformation usually require dimensional data, and since most clinical indexes contain non-dimensional data, the transfers are seldom encountered in clinimetric activities.

3.7. Statistical Expression of Output Scales

In certain circumstances, the clinimetric index provides an output value that is transformed statistically for its ultimate citation and usage. In the statistical transformations, the original output value can be expressed as a proportion of some other value, or as a summary of a set of repeated values.

3.7.1. PROPORTIONATE EXPRESSIONS

A child's intelligence quotient, although seemingly a single score, is actually a proportionate expression. The value obtained in the intelligence test is divided by the value expected for children of that age, and the resulting quotient is the IQ score. This type of expression is also used in pulmonary function tests when a patient's observed vital capacity is divided by the predicted vital capacity to form an index called *percentage vital capacity*.

The value used as the denominator in these statistical proportions can be an expected score (as in the two examples just cited) or a maximum score. Thus, in an index that expresses the severity of daily pain in a patient with peptic ulcer, the total score of the daily ratings is divided by the maximum score that might have been obtained. The result is called the percent of the maximal obtainable epigastric pain score.[1]

3.7.2. SUMMARY OF REPEATED VALUES

When the same index has been rated on repeated occasions in the same person, the individual ratings may not appear as descriptive data. Instead, the array of values may be cited statistically in a single summary expression, which can be a central value (such as a mean or median) for the array, or a regression (or other appropriate) coefficient for the trend observed in the values. Sometimes the clinimetric values are converted into events, and the summary expression is a citation of the proportion of certain types of events. For example, a patient may keep a diary in which severity of daily pain is rated on a scale of **0, 1, 2, 3, 4**. Ratings of **0, 1,** or **2** may then be deemed as good control and **3** and **4** deemed as poor control. The results may receive a summary expression that is calculated as the proportion of all daily ratings that showed good control.

The summary expression can sometimes be derived as a relatively simple sum of the observed values or of appropriate differences in values. An illustration of this process occurs in the *Sum of Pain Intensity Differences* (SPID) *Score* used in studies of analgesic agents.[66] As noted in the title of the score, the patient's intensity of pain is rated on different occasions after treatment. On each occasion, a decrement (or increment) is determined between the original rating and the current rating. The sum of these decrements becomes the SPID score. It is a separate clinimetric variable, obtained as a statistical summary of ratings for the primary clinimetric index, which is *Intensity of Pain.* A somewhat analogous statistical process is used when the diagnosis of diabetes mellitus is established according to the sum of values in a glucose tolerance test.[125]

In the examples just cited, the statistical summary expression gave an individual result that became a separate clinimetric index for each person. Occasionally, however, a set of repeated observations for a *group* of people may be converted into a summary expression for the entire group. This group expression may then become the prime index used in the research. For example, in a comparison of two treatments intended to lower serum cholesterol level, a regression coefficient for the time trend of cholesterol values in patients treated with Agent A may be contrasted with the corresponding coefficient for patients treated with Agent B. In this type of situation the treatments are ultimately evaluated not according to the originally measured values of cholesterol, but according to the regression coefficients that summarize the post-therapeutic trend in each group.

Chapter 4

Choice of Component Variables

Before any component variables are combined or given scalar expressions in an index, a great many decisions must be made. The investigator must first form a clear idea of the purpose of the index and the framework in which it will be applied. The next step in the process includes a series of conceptual decisions that precede the choice of candidate variables. For these decisions, the investigator reviews background information, chooses the types of evidence, plans a focus of interpersonal exchange, and identifies the phenomena or "constructs" that are to be addressed by the index. After these decisions are completed, the candidate variables are chosen, examined, and reduced to the ones that are retained as component variables.

This chapter is concerned with the various forms of strategy used for these decisions. Although clinicians can use the strategies directly, particularly for relatively simple indexes, an additional strategic approach involves the solicitation of advice and guidance from psychosocial scientists who are experts in -metric activities. This type of collaboration is often sought for constructing complex composite indexes, particularly when the indexes deal with disability, functional capacity, health status, satisfaction, or psychosocial features of human life. The collaboration is often highly successful, but it sometimes leads to unhappy results if the psychosocial experts approach the work with conceptual backgrounds and goals that differ substantially from those of the medical clinicians, and if the unrecognized differences lead to major deviations from the basic clinical purposes of the index.

The discussion that follows is divided into three main parts: the conceptual background for an index, the selection of candidate variables, and the decisions about the important candidates that will be retained as component variables. Because many of these activities are often approached differently by clinicians and by psychosocial scientists, the differences will be noted, when pertinent, throughout the discussion. The purpose of citing the differences is to allow both the clinical and the psychosocial collaborators to have a better understanding of one another's approaches, and also to make clinicians aware of alternative strategies that may sometimes be better (or worse) than the customary clinical procedures.

4.1. Conceptual Background

The conceptual background for selection of candidate variables includes at least four activities that can occur in various sequences. In the presentation here, the first step is a review of background information, followed by a consideration of the types of evidence to be included in the index. Next comes a choice of the focus of interpersonal exchange. The fourth step, which can sometimes come first, is an identification of the phenomena or "constructs" that are either described or created by the index.

4.1.1. REVIEW OF BACKGROUND INFORMATION

In choosing the particular variables to include in an index, the investigator can work empirically from a background of documentary data if specific information is available to show the actual effect of each variable in the role for which it is proposed. For example, if persuasive data show that men and women have substantially different rates of outcome for a particular clinical condition, gender might be chosen as a component variable in a prognostic index. If the outcome rates are similar, gender might be eliminated from further consideration.

If no empirical data are available, the background information for choosing candidate variables usually consists of traditional custom, conventional wisdom, personal experience, or some other form of judgment as a guide to what is important. In the traditional-custom approach, the investigator uses the variables that have been emphasized, without documentary evidence, in published literature about the phenomena under study. In the conventional-wisdom approach, the investigator relies on general (although often unpublished) beliefs of the clinical community. In the personal-experience approach, investigators review their own previous clinical adventures to recall what seemed most important. Other sources of judgment involve the assembly of groups of colleagues or authorities who attempt to reach consensual agreement about the decisions. Such methods as the *Nominal Group* and *Delphi techniques* can be used to obtain a consensus.[64]

Different patterns of professional behavior create major differences in the background information available to clinicians and to psychosocial scientists. A psychosocial investigator usually sees the research subject once, while the research is being done; the main data under consideration are obtained primarily from the research questionnaire or instrument. Clinicians, on the other hand, see patients repeatedly over a short or long period of time, collecting many additional forms of data, which may help identify, emphasize, and verify the observed entity.

The additional information can come from at least four different sources. One source is concomitant clinical observation of other phenomena. For example, a patient's report of excruciating pain would not be credible if the patient seems placid and undistressed while the pain is occurring. A second source of additional data is concomitant laboratory information, such as a hematocrit measurement that confirms a clinical observation of pallor and diagnosis of anemia. A third type of additional or validating data can come from the patient's family or other sources of statements that can indicate or verify previous exposure to occupational, pharmaceutical, or other agents. Finally, important data can come from observation of the patient's later clinical course. For example, because histologic evidence is usually too inconvenient or hazardous to be obtained routinely, a diagnosis of acute pancreatitis is usually confirmed by an appropriate set of events and timing in the patient's subsequent state.

This type of additional information gives medical clinicians a great deal of useful background evidence that is seldom available in psychosocial research. The extra information augments and expands the data base clinicians can use to choose and evaluate candidate variables.

4.1.2. INTRINSIC OR EXTRINSIC FOCUS OF EVIDENCE

The type of evidence used to describe a particular phenomenon can be intrinsic or extrinsic. The evidence is *intrinsic* (or "proximal") if it is a direct description of the observed phenomenon. For example, the pain of angina pectoris is described with intrinsic information if a patient reports the location, mode of provocation, frequency, duration, quality, and other characteristics of the pain. For congestive heart failure, the intrinsic information might contain an account of hypertrophy, dilatation, ventricular function, or other things that are happening in the heart itself. The evidence is *extrinsic* (or "distal") if it reflects a consequence or indirect effect of the observed phenomenon. When a patient describes the functional effects that angina pectoris or congestive heart failure have produced in his occupational capacity and life style, the information is extrinsic.

Extrinsic evidence can have at least three different levels of separation from the proximal phenomenon. At the first level, the evidence reflects an immediate although indirect consequence of the phenomenon. Thus, because direct cardiac evidence is seldom observed clinically, congestive heart failure is usually described with extrinsic clinical evidence, manifested by the immediate consequences in the lungs, liver, extremities, neck veins, or other sites elsewhere in the body outside the heart.

At the second level of extrinsic separation, the evidence reflects a patient's subjective response or reaction to the first-level consequences. Such evidence is provided by information about the impact of the congestive failure on the patient's functional capacity in various activities of daily life. At the third level of separation, the extrinsic evidence reflects the way that someone else responds or reacts to the phenomena observed in the patient. Thus, the severity of congestive heart failure might be described according to a clinician's actions in prescribing treatments or arranging hospitalization.

The ability to achieve a standardized rating scale will often depend on the intensity of the subjective decisions needed to provide the intrinsic or extrinsic evidence. For example, we may have difficulty establishing or determining the subjective criteria for rating an anginal pain intrinsically as mild or severe, but we can readily standardize a scale for extrinsic, apparently objective evidence about occupational capacity or supplemental use of nitroglycerine tablets.

In ordinary clinical practice, clinicians will often use direct intrinsic evidence whenever possible, despite the absence of standardized ratings. The direct data can readily be corroborated (as discussed later) by many other forms of information, and the intrinsic phenomenon is often the main focus of pharmacologic or other therapy. This emphasis on intrinsic evidence may then lead to accusations that clinicians have neglected important extrinsic evidence about functional consequences. For example, in cancer chemotherapy, the effects of treatment are usually appraised from direct intrinsic evidence on shrinkage or other changes in the tumor, with lesser attention given to extrinsic information about the patient's relief of symptoms, functional status, and quality of life.

In psychosocial research, direct intrinsic evidence is difficult both to standardize and to confirm. Thus, if we ask a person to rate his degree of ethnic prejudice on a visual analog scale, or in categories such as **none, slight, moderate, or considerable,** we do not know what the person uses as criteria for the ratings, and we may have no way of checking them. To avoid these problems, psychosocial scientists often seek extrinsic evidence, which can be more easily checked and organized into a standard scale. Ethnic prejudice might thus be rated extrinsically according to the patient's responses to diverse ethnic situations—such as willingness to have an ethnic person as a coworker, neighbor, friend, or spouse—that may occur in daily life.

4.1.3. TYPE OF INTERPERSONAL EXCHANGE

In medical practice, patients are accustomed to providing highly intimate personal information. They will usually anticipate and willingly answer questions about defecation, urination, sexual activity, other body functions, and various personal habits and feelings that would be regarded as too private for discussion in almost any other form of discourse between a client and a professional consultant. Patients will also readily describe various pains, discomforts, anxieties, and other distresses that are expected and accepted as information to be exchanged in the doctor-patient relationship.

This relationship, which is a unique feature of medical practice, enables clinicians and patients to communicate in a direct personal manner. Clinicians constantly ask questions that are aimed directly at the individual patient, and patients are usually prepared to answer the questions directly. The patients expect that the answers will be kept confidential, received without moralistic appraisal, and used to plan the specific beneficial actions of the clinician's "samaritan" function.[115]

This type of intimate, personal interchange between investigator and subject seldom occurs when information is collected in psychosocial research. To avoid invading personal privacy and to allow answers whose candor is free of the fears of moral or ethical opprobrium, the psychosocial questions may often be asked in a much more impersonal, indirect manner than would occur in medical communication. Psychosocial comments may be solicited about general appraisals, such as "How do you think most people feel about this?", rather than individual reactions, such as "How do *you* feel about this?" For example, a clinician wanting to know about a patient's attitude toward the hospital's nursing staff might ask, "Are you pleased with the nurses here?" A psychosocial scientist may elicit this information by asking the patient to agree or disagree with a statement such as "Most people are pleased with their nursing care."

The impersonal approach is not always used in psychosocial indexes but has often been advocated for eliciting individual attitudes. The idea is that someone who might be embarrassed or inhibited about openly expressing an unpopular viewpoint may be willing to do so if the attitude can be ascribed to the public at large. Thus, a patient who may not want to hurt the doctor's (or nurse's) feelings by openly stating his own dissatisfaction with care may be willing to express it by saying that most other people are dissatisfied.

Whatever the merits of the impersonal approach, it has the major disadvantage that the respondent may indeed cite general public attitudes rather than individual personal beliefs. A patient who is discontented with his own nursing care may nevertheless answer the general question accurately by stating that most other people are pleased, and the patient's individual opinion may thereby be undetected. Another disadvantage of the impersonal approach is that the avoidance of a direct frontal assault on the target may sometimes lead to an indirect object rather than an indirect subject for the questions. For example, instead of being asked the desired question about satisfaction with nursing care, the patient might be asked to comment on the nurses' uniforms, physical appearance, or other attributes that are tangential to issues in direct care. These comments might elicit the patient's own personal opinion, but not about the main objective of the question.

Major advantages of the medical clinician's highly personal approach are that it focuses specifically on the individual patient, and it allows many questions to be asked and answered in a simple direct manner. The impersonal approach may have certain advantages in getting data about personal attitudes and opinions, but unless the investigators are suitably cautious, the approach may elicit information that is too general or too tangential for achieving the desired goal.

4.1.4. IDENTIFICATION OF PHENOMENA AND 'CONSTRUCTS'

Many of the ideas used in clinical practice refer to intellectual concepts—which psychosocial scientists call "constructs"—that do not exist in tangible form. We cannot actually see, feel, hear, or touch such constructs as congestive heart failure, hepatorenal syndrome, constipation, rheumatic fever, or functional bowel distress. Nevertheless, those constructs are well established and well accepted clinically as pathophysiologic entities or diseases. Other well-established constructs are used when clinicians refer to magnitudes of pain, severity of illness, effects of co-morbidity, or degrees of functional incapacity. If indexes are developed to denote the existence or gradation of these entities, someone may want to quarrel about how well the indexes do their job, but no one will have to be persuaded that the constructs actually exist. For example, some people may not like the New York Heart Association classification of functional incapacity,[24] but functional capacity itself is readily accepted as an entity that warrants classification.

Many of the ideas expressed with psychosocial indexes are also intangible constructs. There is no tangible way to show such constructs as intelligence, familial inter-relationships, maternal-child bonding, or ethnic prejudice. Yet almost everyone, even when dissenting about a proposed method of measurement, will agree that the constructs actually exist. For example, despite many dissatisfactions[70] with the particular techniques used for measuring intelligence, no one would seriously argue against the existence of an entity that could be regarded as intelligence.

Other types of psychosocial constructs, however, are not readily apparent as specific features observed in human behavior. Instead, the constructs are proposed as explanations for certain aggregates of data or variables that emerge from a mathematical analysis. For example, a particular aggregate of weighted variables produced by a factor analysis might be called a right-brain dominant factor, a stress-tension-inward-hostility factor, or a principal component of general intelligence.[70] Being a mathematical product of data analysis, rather than entities identified by direct observation or pathophysiologic conceptualization, these constructs may not always be greeted enthusiastically when first proposed. The investigator may then need to prove that the constructs actually exist and that they have been properly identified as conceptual entities.

For most of the constructs that appear in clinical (and in many psychosocial) indexes, the main challenge is to get a measured description of the idea, not to prove that it exists. In getting an adequate description for an established idea, clinicians can begin immediately with the background information that is already available and can use it directly to select a relatively small number of cogent candidate variables. Psychosocial scientists, on the other hand, may lack suitable background information or may be reluctant to make decisions about cogency without examining a large array of candidates.

4.2. Selection of Candidate Variables

Background information and a knowledge of constructs can act as advantages and disadvantages when a composite index is constructed. Clinicians can easily choose candidate variables for their known cogency without going through a long list of possibilities, but important candidates may be neglected if they are not already expressed in suitable clinimetric scales. Psychosocial scientists may have to examine a long list of candidates, but are not likely to ignore candidates that lack a previous set of suitable scalar expressions.

4.2.1. CLINICAL AND PSYCHOSOCIAL SEQUENCE IN SELECTION

In choosing the cogent variables to be included in an index, clinicians often begin with a clearly observed entity, such as the condition of a newborn baby, that may be cited either with no specific expression or with a global rating, such as **good** or **fair.** The clinimetric activity—as exemplified by the work done when Virginia Apgar created the score now used for this entity—consists of "dissecting" the observed phenomenon or the global rating into its most cogent constituents. For this activity, the clinician reviews his background information with judgmental "intuition" about which observations seem most important. They are then arranged into the axes and variables that form the components of the index.

The psychosocial process, however, often goes in the opposite direction. The most cogent variables emerge after, rather than before, the analysis of assembled data. A psychosocial scientist often begins by collecting a large pool of items, which are individual statements that seem pertinent for the phenomenon under investigation. The pool contains a deliberately excessive number of statements, which will then be appraised and condensed to the particular collection eventually included in the index. The condensation process, as discussed later in Chapter 9, depends on the results found when the statements receive responses from a series of "judges" other than the investigator. The investigator may apply experience and judgment in choosing the original items, reviewing the responses, deciding which ones to retain, putting them together, and labeling the results—but the fundamental decisions about the statements depend on the data provided by the external judges and on the particular theoretical model that was used in reviewing the data.

To illustrate the contrast, the Apgar Score contains the five variables (heart rate, respiratory rate, color, etc.) that were initially chosen by Virginia Apgar as the most cogent descriptions of a newborn baby's condition. A psychosocial index for describing a patient's satisfaction with medical care may contain 40 items that were retained after 100 initial items were rated by a set of judges, with 60 items being eliminated according to certain theoretical principles. Sometimes, in the more complex process discussed in Chapter 8, the retained items are examined further with a mathematical model, such as factor analysis, that aggregates collections of items into special factors. The smaller set of items included in these factors may then be saved in the final citation of the index, and the rest of the items, which did not contribute to the factors, may be eliminated.

In actual operation, therefore, the cogent components of an index can be either identified before the index is constructed, or selected afterward from what was found during the analytic process. In the absence of specific names for these two options, they can be called *dissected intuition* and analytic selection.

4.2.1.1. *Dissected Intuition*

In all the clinimetric examples that have been cited up to now, an index's component variables were derived from the operational policy of dissected intuition. Having repeatedly observed a particular phenomenon and noted various important things about it, most clinicians usually incorporate the cogent observations as part of intuition or judgment. When asked to specify the cogent elements, the clinician tries to dissect and extricate them from the intellectual matrix in which they have been imbedded. Thus, in formulating a clinical index to describe congestive heart failure, a clinician might think about many different clinical phenomena, but might eventually choose dyspnea and edema as the two most cogent manifestations.

The dissection of intuition to choose cogent manifestations is not always easy. In ordinary clinical practice, a clinician who says that a patient is **improved** seldom stipulates the particular observations that were used for the decision. When the stipulations are sought, the clinician may claim they are too intuitive to be specified. Nevertheless, when further prodded to provide the specifications, the clinician may finally dissect the intuition and note that it was based on changes in such variables as facial appearance, posture in bed, pain, ease of breathing, appetite, or pattern of conversation.

The strategy of dissected intuition is constantly used to create new indexes in clinical medicine. From the judgmental intuition obtained via previous observations, experience, and other sources of information, the clinician tries to identify the particular variables (or axes) that seem most important, and then incorporates the variables or axes directly into the index.

4.2.1.2. *Analytic Selection*

In the basic operational policy for creating psychosocial indexes, the investigator seldom begins with a previously observed set of cogent axes or variables. Instead, working in a reverse direction, the investigator first chooses a set of elemental statements, called *items*, that are believed to have a relationship to the phenomenon under study. The individual items may be chosen with acts of dissected intuition, but no pre-conceived judgments are made about their relative importance, which is to be decided later from analysis of the ratings supplied for the items by a group of selected judges.

The analysis involves a set of theoretical principles that are used to eliminate some of the original items and to preserve others, from which the components and scoring system of the output scale are prepared. An important criterion in those theoretical principles is that the retained items must have received consistent agreement in the judges' ratings. Consequently, the retained items—having been selected for statistical consistency rather than clinical sensibility*—may not necessarily be the ones the investigator regards as the most important attributes of the phenomenon under consideration. (This same type of problem can also occur in clinimetric indexes. For example, the duration of a patient's stay in the hospital may be chosen as an index of quality of health care because length of stay can be determined in a consistent standard way, not because it is a major element in quality of care.)

---

*This is the first of many appearances in this book for the words *sensibility* or *sensible*. They often refer to emotional awareness or physical perception (such as "insensible perspiration"). They also are used in common jargon, however, to mean "having good sense or judgment," as in the phrase "He is a sensible person. He agrees with me." I doubt that my common-jargon meaning will confuse any medical readers, who regularly use (or abuse) *sensible* and *sensibility* in this same way. The possible ambiguity might be avoided if the noun were *sensibleness*, but it is an unfamiliar term and might create confusion rather than clarification. Besides, the *-ity* ending is an attractive linguistic companion for the statistical ideas of *reliability* and *validity* with which clinical sensibility will often be compared. Finally, the other meanings of *sensibility* will usually also be pertinent. In other words, a *sensible* index will seem to "make good sense" if it is suitably aware and perceptive of what it describes.

Judgment is also relegated to mathematical analysis of the data if the investigators examine the results in search of a common theoretical background for individual items in the index. In clinical work, this type of coherence is identified with clinical judgments about biologic plausibility or pathophysiologic explanations. In psychosocial indexes, the coherence is often sought—as discussed in Chapter 8—with mathematical models that assign weighted coefficients to the items and arrange them into additive combinations called factors or principal components. These entities, which are mathematically synthesized after the research is done, then become a counterpart of the axes selected beforehand in the dissected-intuition approach.

Statisticians have sometimes quarreled about the mathematical principles used in factor analysis and principal component analysis, but the results have been well accepted by psychosocial investigators. The method is also sometimes used in matters familiar to medical readers. The mathematical models have produced such things as the Hamilton scale for rating depression,[80] the Type A and Type B patterns of personality traits,[68] a classification of nutritional status,[75] and an index of activity for rheumatic disease.[143]

The methods of analytic selection seem quite reasonable for the task of creating attitude scales for political, social, or psychologic beliefs. In probing a person's attitudinal opinions, an investigator who begins with preconceptions of what is important may merely buttress his own prejudices rather than determine what the person really believes. Therefore, a policy that encourages a free expression of attitudes and that later determines which items are most valuable seems well suited for the goal of creating attitudinal scales. The additional mathematical methods used to investigate coherence of items also seem quite reasonable when a suitable background of observation is not available to provide judgment about the importance or relationships of the variables.

4.2.1.3. *Comparison of the Two Approaches*

Although clinical and psychosocial investigators can be well justified in their separate use of judgmental or mathematical strategies for choosing cogent variables, the strategies are quite different, and those that work well in one domain may not do so in the other. Since the dissected-intuition and analytic-selection options have seldom been deliberately compared in application to the same challenge, neither one can claim superiority. The analytic-selection approach seems appropriate when applied to the study of psychosocial attitudes for which no particular etiologic, diagnostic, prognostic, or therapeutic correlations are available. The dissected-intuition approach seems appropriate for studying clinical phenomena where the correlations obtained during antecedent clinical experience can be effective guides to the choice of important variables.

The main conflicts arise in the cross-over situations, where indexes for clinical phenomena have been created with the mathematical or psychosocial models of analytic selection. Are nutritional status and rheumatic activity better defined by a knowledgeable clinician's dissected intuitions or by a mathematical selection of individual items? Is a clinical attitude, such as patient satisfaction, best determined from a factor analysis of 100 items, or from the simpler scale that might be created if clinicians dissected their observations of satisfied and dissatisfied patients, and developed an appropriate index more directly?

Regardless of what answers are given to these questions, the main point to be noted now is that clinical and psychosocial scientists frequently use different policies. Clinicians often select cogent variables by dissecting their previous intuitions or global observations of a phenomenon whose attributes are directly reflected (or correlated) in the selected variables. Psychosocial scientists often begin with a list of multiple items from which cogent variables are later chosen with theoretical principles of organization and aggregation.

4.2.2. PROBLEMS IN CHOICE OF CLINICAL VARIABLES

When choosing candidate variables, an investigator usually begins by thinking about things that have already been expressed in a suitable format with a delineated scale of categories. If the decision depends on empirical evidence, the scale of categories has already been developed and was used when the data were assembled. Such variables can readily become candidates for inclusion in a composite index.

Many important clinical phenomena, however, may not be overtly available as candidate variables because they have not yet received a specific clinimetric citation. When these phenomena are recognized during judgmental appraisals, the investigator must decide what to do about them. To be included in the "larger" clinimetric index, the phenomena must first receive the "smaller" attention that will make them variables by giving them suitable indexes of their own. If the investigator, aiming at the larger goal, does not take the time and effort needed to construct the additional new indexes, important clinical phenomena may be omitted from the composite expression.

For example, in preparing a composite index to estimate prognosis in patients with cancer, an investigator can readily contemplate such candidate variables as age, gender, hematocrit, primary site of cancer, anatomic spread, and histologic type, because each of these six variables has a distinct method of clinimetric expression. None of these six variables, however, accounts for such prognostically cogent phenomena as clinical severity of illness, comorbidity, and rate of disease progression. If the latter three variables have not been categorized clinimetrically, an investigator who wants to develop an effective prognostic index must first form the new clinimetric indexes that will make the cogent clinical phenomena available as component variables.

The neglect of this challenge has led to some major problems in the current state of clinimetrics. The problems arise not because of difficulties in choosing or combining the existing candidate variables but because important candidates, having no clinimetric indexes of their own, are omitted from consideration.[59]

4.3. Decisions about Importance

From the myriads of variables that can be regarded as appropriate candidates for a particular index, the investigator must choose the ones that are important enough to be included as its components.

4.3.1. COMPETING GOALS IN BASIC DECISIONS

The decision about what is important is a complex act of judgment, which depends on fundamental policy decisions, often involving a choice among several desirable but competing goals that cannot all be attained. The way the investigator assigns priorities to these goals, at a very early phase of the work, will often determine how everything else is done, and how successfully the index fulfills its intended purpose and functional role.

The competition of different goals can be illustrated if we consider the two desiderata of getting an index that is both easy to use and effective. To make the index easy to use, we would want it to contain relatively few component variables; but to let the index do its job effectively, we do not want any potentially important variables to be omitted. If the phenomenon under study requires a consideration of many different variables, we may not easily be able to reduce them to a relatively small collection. We can keep them all and take the risk of having a complicated index that is hard to use but effective; or we can eliminate some of the variables that seem less cogent, taking the risk of an inefficient index that is easy to use.

The best compromise, of course, is to select a relatively small number of variables while including all the ones that are important. This compromise may or may not be successful—but its evaluation will often depend on other basic policy decisions about what attributes should be emphasized to regard an index as successful. Will we be happy if its results are sensible but non-reproducible and inaccurate, or if the results are reproducible and accurate but not sensible? And if we cannot achieve all three of the desired attributes, which ones should be given lesser emphasis, and how much can the emphasis be lowered without creating fatal flaws in the results?

The answers to these questions establish the style of the fundamental scientific policies used in constructing and evaluating an index. Because the style and the policies may differ substantially among the statisticians, psychosocial consultants, and clinicians who often collaborate to form clinimetric indexes, Chapters 8 and 9 will contain an extensive discussion of the basic interdisciplinary differences in -metric goals. For the moment, we can simply note that these differences may lead to disparate standards for evaluating the success of an index, as well as disparate methods for deciding about the importance of variables. Those methods will be briefly outlined here, in preparation for more detailed discussion in Chapters 8 and 9.

4.3.2. METHODS OF DETERMINING IMPORTANCE

The three main methods for determining the importance of variables are clinical judgment, mathematical models, or a combined form of clinico-statistical judgment.

4.3.2.1. *Clinical Judgment*

Decisions about which variables are important in a particular situation can be made with any of the types of clinical judgment, discussed in Section 4.1.1, that rely on traditional custom, conventional wisdom, personal experience, or a consensus of authorities. Being purely judgmental, the strategies will choose the variables that are regarded as important and will omit the others. After these variables have been chosen, they can later be subjected to empirical tests (to be discussed in Chapter 11) that might demonstrate the value of the choices—but the original selections are made without empirical evidence.

A different type of judgment is needed for certain indexes (to be discussed in Chapter 6) that require the active collaboration of patients. When the component variables involve such issues as satisfaction, functional capacity, or quality of life, the best indication of importance is usually obtained from the preferences expressed by the patients themselves, not from judgments made by individual clinicians or by panels of authorities.

4.3.2.2. *Mathematical Models*

At the other end of the decision-making spectrum is a strategy that relies entirely on mathematical models to indicate the relative importance and weight of component variables. In contrast to purely judgmental strategies, which can be applied even when no background data are available, mathematical models require an analysis of empirical evidence.

The choice of models depends on the purpose of their application, the type of available evidence, and the type of output scale that is desired. Thus, the models can be used exclusively for screening the importance of variables, or the output scale can be formed directly as a mathematically prepared aggregate. The evidence can be arranged in a dependent or interdependent manner, and the mathematical output can be an arithmetical score or a Boolean cluster.

Because the operational tactics of the mathematical models will be discussed further in Chapter 8, the only point to be emphasized now is that all these models rely on arbitrary decisions, which involve mathematical rather than clinical or biologic considerations. After arranging to fit the data with a mathematical structure that is conceived as a straight line, plane, multi-dimensional surface, or other spatial configuration, each model usually determines the importance of each variable by noting the impact of that variable on the statistical variance of the data fitted with the model. The only acts of biologic judgment in the mathematical procedures are the original choices of candidate variables that will be entered into the model, and the original decision about expressing the output scale as a score or cluster. Everything else thereafter will depend on the particular mathematical attributes of the selected model, on the arbitrary magnitude chosen to demarcate an important reduction in statistical variance, and on the idiosyncrasies of whatever occurs statistically when the particular collection of data is processed through the selected model.

4.3.2.3. *Clinico-Statistical Judgment*

To avoid the extremes of either clinical judgments that have no confirmatory evidence or mathematical models that have no corroborative judgment, a combined form of strategy can be used. For example, certain prognostic indexes have been constructed as clusters of categories that were originally chosen according to clinical judgment, but aggregated according to their statistical effects on the outcome that is being predicted.[47] The aggregation would be arranged to form a distinct prognostic gradient for the clustered ordinal categories of the scale. Additional variables, beyond those already incorporated in the index, would show their prognostic importance by creating new gradients within the previous array of gradients. This double-gradient phenomenon reduces variance in the data for clustered categories and is analogous to the other measurements of variance reduction that are used to determine the importance of variables in conventional mathematical models. When the clustered categories are formed with clinico-statistical judgment, the investigator uses empirical data to provide statistical evidence for the value of all decisions that combine categories, but the decisions are made in a sequence of steps each of which is checked for its sensibility according to clinical judgment.

A type of clinico-statistical judgment is also used in psychosocial strategy when the candidate items for an index are submitted for responses by a panel of judges, who need not be experts and who are often the same kind of persons to whom the developed index will later be applied. The ratings of the judges are used to reduce the original list of statements to a smaller important group, but the items retained as constituents of the index may first be required to show statistical evidence of consistency in the judges' responses.

4.4. **Stipulation of Component Variables**

Regardless of how the component variables are chosen, they must be suitably identified for reproducible usage. This issue in basic stipulation creates some of the most obvious and widespread problems in clinimetric indexes. The component variables may not be identified at all, or their rating scale may not be listed, or the categories of the scale may be cited without criteria for demarcation.

The problems of reproducible identification are somewhat analogous to those of providing an adequate recipe in cooking. For certain cooks, an instruction such as "heat until the liquid is hot enough" will be clear. Other cooks may want greater detail such as "heat until the liquid boils." Yet other cooks may want criteria that indicate how to recognize and decide that a liquid is boiling. Someone who has never done any cooking may also want to know what type of container to put the liquid in, what type of heat to apply, and how much time the heating process might take.

Except for global scales concerned with complex phenomena, the component variables of a composite index are almost always identified by a name or title. The main problems in stipulation occur if the titular name does not clearly indicate what it refers to. For example, if severity of diarrhea is a component variable in an index, what aspect of the diarrhea is to be evaluated for severity? Frequency, pain, texture of stools, impact on daily life, or other features?

Because different users of an index will need or want different degrees of detail, standards cannot readily be established for suitability in the recipe that stipulates the operation of the index. We can get a good idea of what should be covered, however, if we recall that an index is created by identifying components, combining those components into axes, and combining the axes into the output scale. We shall therefore need to identify each of the component variables and its scale of citation. If axes are used, we need to identify the rating scale for each axis and the mechanism by which component parts are aggregated in the axis. Finally, we need to identify the output scale and the way that the axes or basic components are aggregated to form that scale.

The structure of the output scale, which is a particularly critical feature of composite indexes, will be discussed in the next chapter.

Chapter 5

Organization of the Output Scale

After being chosen and stipulated, the components of a composite index are converted into a set of categories that constitute the output scale. Although the results of this scale become the main data that are used in subsequent interpretations and analyses of the index, the underlying adequacy of the output scale depends on how well it was organized. The organization, which is discussed in this chapter, requires that the component categories be suitably arranged and that the arrangement be suitably stipulated.

A suitable arrangement for an output scale depends on the scope, discrimination, and coherence of its categories. The first two attributes— scope and discrimination—can usually be appraised without any deep knowledge or consideration of the scientific entity to which the scale refers. With a simple examination of the available categories, a thoughtful person should be able to determine whether the output scale will have suitable scope and discrimination.

For example, a scale that offers **doctor** and **lawyer** as its only categories would obviously have an unsuitable scope for specifying occupation. A thermometer that has markings only at **37, 38,** and **39°C** would have unsuitable discrimination for specifying temperature. Although these issues in scope and discrimination can often be easily discerned, a simple inspection of the contents of the scale will not suffice to appraise its coherence, which depends on the scientific connotation of the categories and the purpose for which they are used.

These issues in scope, discrimination, and coherence seldom create substantial problems in the formation and evaluation of laboratory measurements. If we set up a mechanism to measure the quantitative concentration of serum molybdenum, we would want to have suitable scope in covering the range of possible values, and suitable discrimination in isolating molybdenum and in distinguishing different magnitudes of concentration. These two desiderata are relatively easy to determine; and if they cannot be achieved, we would search for a different mechanism of measurement. When the mechanism is finally chosen, however, we would not have to worry about problems of coherence in deciding whether the scale of measurement should be expressed differently for diagnostic or prognostic purposes. We also need not fear that we might have inappropriately combined molybdenum, cholesterol, and sodium into a single expression.

All of these problems can create major obstacles or defects when several component variables are joined in the composite scales constructed as clinimetric indexes. Inadequacies in scope and discrimination can occur without being promptly recognized; and the evaluation of coherence for multiple variables involves judgments that are not required in laboratory measurements of single variables.

5.1. Scope of Scale

For a scale to have suitable scope, the categories should fully cover the range of possible expressions, should be mutually exclusive of one another but exhaustively inclusive for the component parts, and should have realistic values. (The discussion that follows is directed at the output scale of a composite index, but the comments will often be equally pertinent for the scale of a single component variable or axis.)

5.1.1. EXHAUSTIVE SCOPE OF CATEGORIES

Suppose we arrange a scale in which political preference is expressed as one of the two binary categories, **Democratic** or **Republican.** Such a scale is non-exhaustive because it contains no categories with which to list a person who is **undecided** or who prefers some other political party.

Concern about an exhaustive range of categories is seldom a prominent problem in laboratory forms of measurement because the scale of a dimensional variable usually has no fixed limits and can readily expand its range to cover the observed magnitudes. Even if a particular value is outside the range of measurement on an existing scale, the result can be cited as below the lowest or above the highest category in the scale. Thus, if we cannot accurately measure serum glucose values that are below 40 or above 1000 mgm/dl, we can always use such expressions as **<40** or **>1000;** or we can change to a more precise mechanism for measuring the extremely low or high values.

In the nominal or binary categories of a clinimetric scale, however, this type of beyond-the-boundary expression cannot be readily applied. We cannot rate a person's political preference as being "higher" than **Democratic** or "lower" than **Republican.** Accordingly, the scope of categories requires special attention in clinimetric scales. An easy way to take care of the problem of scope is always to include such categories as **other, unknown** (used when no data exist), and **uncertain** (used when information is available but is not precise enough to allow assignment of any of the available categories). Although this mechanism would solve the problem of scope, it would not allow suitable discrimination if we wanted to know the particular preferences cited in the category of **other.**

A special challenge in certain types of ordinal ratings involves the decision to include or exclude a neutral category. Suppose we want to indicate whether a patient has or has not had an acute myocardial infarction. If the scale is constructed with four categories—**definitely yes, probably yes, probably no, definitely no**—the diagnosis will be rated as positive or negative for each patient, but if the scale includes **"uncertain whether yes or no"** as a fifth neutral category in the middle of the scale, many patients may be given that rating. Because the inclusion or omission of a neutral category can produce crucial changes in results, the decision will depend on the particular goals of the research or other uses of the data.[94,129]

5.1.2. MUTUALLY EXCLUSIVE CATEGORIES

A scale will create ambiguity if it contains two or more categories that are not mutually exclusive. For example, suppose a scale for patient's chief complaint contains the categories **fever, fatigue, pain,** and **other.** The scale is exhaustive because the category of **other** can be used for any chief complaint that is not fever, fatigue, or pain. The scale is ambiguous, however, because we would not know which category to use for classifying a patient whose chief complaint is both fever and fatigue, fever and pain, all three symptoms, or combinations of one of those symptoms and something else.

This problem, which is particularly likely to occur with nominal scales, can be managed by listing each possible combination as an individual category, e.g., **fever alone, fatigue alone, fever and fatigue, pain alone, fever and pain,** etc. An often better approach, however, is to convert the nominal categories to binary variables in separate scales. In the example here, the new array of four variables would have scales of **yes** or **no** for *fever* as one variable, for *fatigue* as another variable, for *pain,* and for *other.* If one (or more) of these four entities must be designated as the *chief complaint,* a special coding can be used for the designation, but the presence of the other symptoms would also be noted appropriately.[40]

An undesirable approach is to force the user of the overlapping categories in the single scale to select only one of them as the chief complaint. If the patient's chief complaint is the combination of fever and fatigue, the single-choice approach will lead to a loss of important information and to distortions in the subsequent results. (The exclusionary procedure, unfortunately, is used throughout the world by health agencies that deal with death certificates. Of the many diseases that may have contributed to a patient's death, only one is permitted to be listed as *the* single cause of death. The inconsistency with which the single-cause choices are made both by practicing clinicians and by statistical coders at the health agencies is a prominent source of the defects in national and international data tabulated as "cause-specific mortality" from death certificates.)[54]

5.1.3. EXHAUSTIVE INCLUSION OF COMPONENTS

Suppose an index contains three component variables, A, B, and C, each of which is scored in a binary rating of **present** or **absent.** The output scale will have to account for eight possible combinations of categories in the three component variables. The arrangement is shown in the Venn diagram of Figure 5.1. In one combination (Sector 1 of the diagram), A, B, and C are all **present;** in another (Sector 2), all three are **absent.** In the remaining arrangements, three (Sectors 3, 4, and 5) will have one of the three variables **present** and the other two **absent;** and the other three arrangements (Sectors 6, 7, and 8) will have one of the three variables **absent** with the other two **present.**

The particular way in which the eight categories are rated depends on their importance and on the goals of the scale—but all eight categories must be accounted for. If the components are not exhaustively included in the output categories, the scale will be difficult to use and the results will be inconsistent.

This type of problem was noted[90] as a source of observer variability in the use of a Performance Status index proposed by Karnofsky.[96] The components of the index depend on **positive** or **negative** ratings for three variables: ability to work, to carry on normal activities without assistance, and to care for personal needs. The eight possible combinations of these binary factors, however, were not all included in the arrangements of the output scale. For example, the scale contains no category with which to cite the state of a paraplegic musician who can work successfully but needs aid in other activities.

5.1.4. REALISTIC VALUES

A scale will have unrealistic values if its components can be arranged to produce categories that are biologically impossible. For example, suppose a

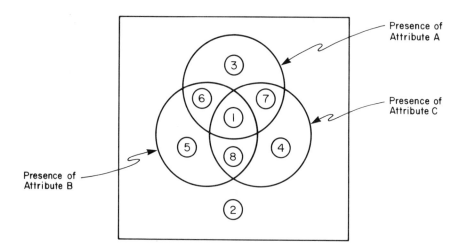

Figure 5.1. Venn diagram showing eight categories formed as combinations of three binary component variables.

composite index is created by combining two binary variables, each expressed as **yes** or **no** for *female gender* and for *presence of pregnancy*. When the first variable is scored as **no** and the second as **yes,** the output scale will denote a pregnant man.

A more pragmatic example of this problem, which is further discussed in Chapter 8, occurs when the scale is an arithmetical score produced by the mathematical model of multiple linear regression. In such a model, expressed as $y = b_0 + b_1x_1 + b_2x_2 + b_3x_3 + \ldots$, the output-scale value for y often represents a probability. Thus, y might be the probability of survival at three years for a particular patient having the values of $x_1, x_2, x_3, \ldots$ that are entered into the regression formula. Because y represents a probability, its results should always be between **0** and **1.** Nevertheless, when data for individual patients are entered into linear regression formulas, the value of y that emerges for probability of survival can sometimes be negatively smaller than 0 or positively greater than 1. To avoid this peculiarity, the multiple linear regression model is often replaced by the multiple logistic regression model, which constrains the results so that the values of y always lie between 0 and 1.

5.2. **Discrimination of Scale**

In dimensional measurements, we may not always want to make the results as precise as possible. Thus, we usually cite an adult's age in years, rather than in months, days, or hours. With a newborn baby, however, we might want to discriminate age more precisely, and we might therefore use hours, days, or weeks as the scale of measurement.

The choice of suitable discrimination is a tricky challenge, which involves a compromise between the needs of the user and the role of the data. If the discrimination is too great, the scale may be difficult to use because the choice of categories is beyond customary human capacities in observation and discernment. If the discrimination is too small, the scale may be easy to use, but important distinctions may be neglected or missed in the data.

5.2.1. EXCESSIVE DISCRIMINATION

When scientific measurements are conventionally reported in three significant digits and percentages are cited in two digits, the customs arise for two reasons. In most instances of measurement, three digits (accompanied if necessary by additional exponents, such as 3.73×10^5 or 8.41×10^{-3}) will suffice to discriminate the magnitude of the results. For most percentages, the human mind can easily remember and evaluate two digits rather than three.[34]

In clinimetric measurements, the problem of excessive discrimination arises when a scale requires discernments that are too difficult to make. Suppose you are asked to use a scale that has the ranked categories of **1, 2, 3, 4, 5,** or **6** for giving a global rating to the auscultatory loudness of a cardiac murmur. Regardless of what criteria you use for these ratings, you can probably develop a reasonable mechanism for deciding when to apply **1** as the lowest value and **6** as the highest value and when to use the intermediate values of **2, 3, 4,** or **5.** If you are asked, instead, to give this same global rating, but using a scale that has **1, 2, 3,...8, 9, 10** as its categories, you might have substantial difficulty (or even discomfort) in making the discernments, but you might eventually develop a reasonably consistent mechanism of discrimination.

Suppose, however, that you were asked to rate the auscultatory loudness of a murmur by using the scale of **1, 2, 3,..., 36, 37, 38,..., 97, 98, 99, 100.** This scale would be impossible to apply in any practical manner. How easily could you decide between a rating of **37** vs. **38**, or **72** vs. **73**? The fine discrimination required in such a scale is beyond our capacity of discernment for the phenomenon under observation. There would be many problems of intra-observer variability when we used the scale repeatedly for our own ratings, and inter-observer variability when we checked agreement for different observers.

This type of difficulty is the reason so many global clinimetric scales are expressed in a limited number of categories, such as **0, 1+, 2+, 3+,** and **4+.** A small group of ratings can be discerned more readily and reproducibly than a larger selection. For example, the global ratings of the Karnofsky Performance Index, which can be expressed either on a quasi-dimensional scale of **0** to **100** or with the ordinal grades of **A, B,** and **C,** were more reproducible when the ratings were cited on the scale with fewer categories.[90]

5.2.2. INADEQUATE DISCRIMINATION

Although a small number of categories is easy to use, the scale may not discriminate well, particularly when employed to detect changes rather than to denote a single status. Such ratings as **A, B,** or **C** may be quite satisfactory for classifying each person's performance status at a single point in time, but at a later date, when we want to discern each person's change, the single-status ratings may not be adequate for showing transitions.

For example, a patient who is essentially confined to bed might initially be rated as **C** in performance status. Later on, the patient may still be confined to bed and may still receive a rating of **C** but may have substantially improved in urinary continence and in the ability to feed himself. The improvement will not be detected, however, if we compare the two status ratings of **C.**

5.2.3. OBSCURE DISCRIMINATION

When a rating is prepared as an aggregate of multiple component variables, the identity, as well as the source, of certain distinctive phenomena may be obscured. For example, if a baby has an Apgar score of **5,** we do not know whether heart rate has been graded as **0, 1,** or **2.** If we merely want to classify the baby's state for a collection of Apgar scores, the rating of **5** may be quite satisfactory. If we want to know specifically about heart rate, however, its condition is obscured in the aggregate score.

The same type of problem arises if the baby's Apgar score is **5** at one minute and **7** at five minutes after birth. The higher score would show that an improvement has occurred, but we cannot determine (if we want to know) which of the five components of the score have improved or whether any have gotten worse.

5.2.4. METHODS OF IMPROVING DISCRIMINATION

The strategies that can be used to increase discrimination depend upon the source of the difficulties.

5.2.4.1. *Increased Number of Categories*

If the output scale is coarse, with too few categories, the number of categories can be increased. Thus, a status scale that contains only three categories can be expanded to include six, seven, or more. This approach is particularly appealing and easy if the additional categories can be readily identified and delineated. With more categories available for the spread of single-state ratings, the scale should be better able to show changes. On the other hand, the increased number of categories may make the scale more difficult to use for its role as a status index. The extra number of categories may produce the excessive-discrimination hazard discussed in Section 5.2.1.

5.2.4.2. *Transition Indexes*

To avoid the hazard just cited, clinimetricians have begun to use an alternative approach, which involves the construction of an additional, separate index of change. Because a status index and a change index have two different roles and may therefore require two different constructions, a separate transition index may often offer a highly effective method of measuring change. With this technique, a patient's functional status (as an example) would be classified with two indexes rather than one. The first would be a single-state index of *functional status*. The second would be a transition index for showing *change in functional status*. The second index would be expressed in a transition scale, such as **substantially improved, slightly improved, no change, slightly worse,** and **substantially worse.** Having a limited number of categories, this scale would be easy to use, and it would obviously discriminate change since it is aimed directly at indicating change.

The development of separate transition indexes is a relatively distinctive activity in clinimetrics because such indexes are seldom needed for the entities described with dimensional data in laboratory or engineering measurements. The processes that can be used to construct separate transition indexes are illustrated in the now traditional scale of ratings for pain relief[66] and in more recent indexes that show changes in the functional state of patients with angina pectoris,[49] changes in the severity of sore-throat pain,[141] or changes in clinical dyspnea.[118]

As a new type of -metric activity, the construction of separate transition indexes offers many intriguing intellectual challenges. They include the selection of optimal formats for the output scale, the desirability of maintaining symmetrical categories for each direction of change,[117] the appraisal of relationships between changes and baseline status, and the possible virtues of eliminating a developed transition scale by incorporating its distinctions into an expanded single-status scale.

5.2.4.3. *Focus on Important Components*

If obscure discrimination is produced by an excess of component variables, the obscurity can be reduced or eliminated by removing the extra component variables. When we want to know mainly about changes in Variable A, the index used to discern the change should focus mainly or exclusively on Variable A, without including Variables B, C, D, and E as additional components. If the A-B-C-D-E combination is valuable as an aggregated index, the aggregate can be preserved for the particular purpose it serves. A separate index (or the subscale for Variable A) can then be used alone for the separate purpose of identifying changes in Variable A.

The main difficulty in this type of procedure is making the decision that Variable A warrants being the focus of attention. The decision, which requires a mechanism for identifying the importance of Variable A, can be approached with any of the strategies noted in Section 4.3.2. Alternatively, as discussed in Chapter 6, the patient's preference can sometimes be solicited to indicate the most important variable(s).

5.3. Coherence of Scale

The scope and discrimination of a scale can readily be evaluated by an intelligent person examining its structure, without any profound knowledge of the particular clinical or scientific phenomena to which the index is addressed. The person may not need to be an expert in anything (other than scale making) to determine that the categories are non-exhaustive, ambiguous, or inadequate for satisfactory discrimination. To appraise the coherence of a scale, however, will usually require special knowledge of the topic and purpose of the index.

5.3.1. BIOMETRIC COHERENCE

The biometric coherence of a scale involves both the biologic and statistical suitability of the aggregated components.

5.3.1.1. *Biologic Plausibility*

When several different variables are aggregated into a composite index, the conjunctions can be examined for the biologic plausibility that justifies combining either the basic variables themselves or the constituent elements that form individual categories in the output scale.

For example, suppose we decide to combine three variables—*severity of symptoms, severity of co-morbidity,* and *favorite hobby*—into a composite index of clinical status for a patient with cancer. No matter how well the output scale is constructed, and no matter how well its categories produce suitable scope and discrimination, the index will not seem biologically plausible because *favorite hobby* is not an appropriate component in an index concerned with *clinical status.* If we omitted *favorite hobby,* however, the other two variables would go together in a plausible manner.

Now suppose that *severity of clinical status* is an index created by joining two binary variables that refer to *cachexia* and *severity of co-morbidity.* Since the combination of these two variables is biologically plausible, we next examine what happens in the output scale. Suppose that *cachexia* is expressed as **absent** or **present,** and that *severity of co-morbidity* has the binary citation of **no decompensation** or **decompensation of major organ system** (such as congestive heart failure, respiratory insufficiency, or hepatic failure). When the categories of these two binary variables are combined, the output scale must account for four possible arrangements. All four arrangements are plausible, since a patient might have both cachexia and decompensation, cachexia without decompensation, decompensation without cachexia, or neither. When we attach names to these four arrangements, the severity of clinical status can quite plausibly be rated as **poor** for someone who has both cachexia and decompensation, but what terms should be used for the other three arrangements? Would we want to rate the status as **good** for someone who has one of these attributes but not the other, and **excellent** for someone who has neither cachexia nor decompensation? Since a patient might also have widespread cancer metastases or repeated episodes of ventricular fibrillation, which are not represented in the composite index, we might be reluctant to rate severity of clinical status as **excellent** merely because cachexia and decompensation are absent. Because either attribute is so undesirable, we also would regard **good** as an unsatisfactory rating for someone who has one of them but not the other.

Evaluations of plausibility will often involve judgments that depend on both scientific knowledge and the particular purpose of the index. In the example just cited, the decision that the index had an unsatisfactory scale depended on clinical knowledge that *severity of clinical status* could be affected by variables other than *cachexia* and *co-morbidity.* As another example, consider a composite index, called *distant metastasis,* that is cited as **present** or **absent** for a patient with cancer of the prostate. The composite index is rated as **present** if a positive value appears for any of three existential variables that express the presence of metastatic *cancer in liver, cancer in brain,* or *cancer in bone.* The three individual variables and the output scale are all quite acceptable as a clinical combination in this index, but the arrangement of these particular variables and the idea of "distant metastasis" would not be satisfactory if the primary site of the cancer were in liver, brain, or bone, rather than prostate.

Beyond these determinations of suitability, the greatest scientific virtue of biologic plausibility is that it can allow a composite index to serve as both a label and an explication for the constituent categories. This type of explication constantly occurs when an index provides a set of diagnostic criteria. For example, the individual existential variables of arthritis, carditis, and chorea appear to refer to three different types of clinical phenomena; but they immediately make sense and become explained when they are combined, using the Jones diagnostic criteria, into a single existential index for presence of rheumatic fever. Similarly, such existential entities as peripheral edema, pulmonary rales, and distended neck veins seem to refer to phenomena in three different parts of the body, but they immediately become plausibly combined and explicated with a diagnosis of congestive heart failure.

Biologic plausibility can be provided by mechanisms other than a diagnostic title. For example, suppose we consider three different diagnoses: recurrent myocardial infarctions, hepatic encephalopathy, and pulmonary decompensation. These three entities cannot be readily joined into a single diagnostic explication, but they are plausibly united into an index that expresses the presence of poor prognosis. An even larger variety of clinical entities could be plausibly listed in the nominal scale of an index referring to conditions that often have a positive response to corticosteroid therapy.

The capacity to form biologically plausible combinations is a uniquely human skill. It cannot be done by a mathematical model or computer program. No matter how ingenious the mathematical strategy or logical algorithm, an inanimate system would not be able to produce the labeled cluster for distant metastasis, rheumatic fever, or congestive heart failure unless the concepts and criteria had previously been entered by a human mind into the automated system.

These human judgments can also be applied for deciding whether to use a score or a cluster arrangement in an output scale. Thus, in forming the score by which she is commemorated, Virginia Apgar chose to make and add numerical ratings for the five component variables rather than trying to form clusters of categories. In other circumstances, however, a cluster may be much more biologically informative than a score, and the clusters may be easier to arrange when derived from component variables that are cited in categorized ratings such as **present** or **absent.** For example, suppose we use the rating scale of **0** or **1** for each of three existential variables that refer to the absence or presence of peripheral edema, pulmonary rales, and distended neck veins. When the composite output scale is prepared by adding the three ratings, the presence of all three clinical manifestations would be scored as a **3.** On the other hand, if we think about the clinical connotation of the three constituent variables, a patient who has **peripheral edema, pulmonary rales,** and **distended neck veins** might be much more informatively categorized with the cluster title of **congestive heart failure.**

Because biologic coherence is relatively easy to evaluate in a clustered category but is more difficult to discern in a score, clinicians usually prefer to express intricate judgments with output scales that contain categories rather than scores. Despite the enormous scientific appeal of a numerical score, dimensional or ranked data are regularly converted into categorical arrangements (such as **abnormal** or **normal, too high** or **too low, presence** or **absence** of Disease D, **use** or **do not use** Treatment T, **too sick** or **not sick enough**) when major clinical decisions are made.

5.3.1.2. *Statistical Isometry*

When we previously combined **recurrent myocardial infarctions, hepatic encephalopathy,** and **pulmonary decompensation** into a single categorical cluster called **poor prognosis,** the combination was justified with purely clinical judgment. We could also, however, test this combination with real-world statistical evidence. Thus, if the one-year survival rates were all similar and very low for patients with any one of the three cited entities, the combination would be statistically *isometric* as well as biologically plausible. On the other hand, if the one-year survival rates were 3% for patients with hepatic encephalopathy, 15% for patients with recurrent myocardial infarctions, and 60% for patients with pulmonary decompensation, the three conditions would not be isometric for their one-year survival rate. They could become isometric, however, if we were concerned with five-year rather than one-year survival, and if patients in each of those three groups had a five-year survival rate of less than 1%.

Unless specific evidence has been checked to confirm the isometry of the elements collected in a cluster, the rational appeal of biologic plausibility may produce combinations that are not statistically coherent. For example, in patients with lung cancer, the cluster category of **distant metastasis** is an attractive way to combine such component categories as presence of **metastasis to brain, metastasis to liver,** and **metastasis to extrathoracic bone.** Nevertheless, the survival rates at brief periods, such as six months, are substantially higher in lung-cancer patients with metastasis to brain than in patients with the other two types of metastasis.[50] If the three types of distant metastasis are combined into a single category, the cluster may be highly coherent and plausible biologically, but the six-month survival results will not make good sense statistically because they combine heterogeneous prognostic phenomena.

A quite different type of statistical isometry is used when the components of an index are joined because they show high correlations with one another rather than with an external target (or dependent) variable. For example, in the previous paragraph, metastases to sites such as brain, liver, and extrathoracic bone were joined in the single category of **distant metastasis** because they had similar correlations with the outcome variable of survival. In other circumstances, however, when the index is formed without an external dependent variable, certain variables may be joined because they show a high interdependent correlation with one another. Thus, if we formed an index without regard to survival outcome, such features as **abnormal brain scan, Babinski sign,** and **paralysis of leg** might be highly intercorrelated.

These interdependent correlations are a prime goal of the mathematical activities used to form indexes according to such non-target-oriented procedures as factor analysis, principal component analysis, and cluster analysis. When the indexes are later applied, the results in different groups can be checked with Cronbach's alpha (or other calculations noted in Chapter 11) to show the statistical intercorrelation of variables.

The main biologic hazard of isometric groupings formed by statistical intercorrelations is that the results of the calculations will depend on the particular kinds of people whose data are entered into the computations. The mathematical consequences may or may not be biologically cogent. Another hazard is that certain variables having the virtue of a high interdependent correlation may actually be redundant rather than important. For example, in a large collection of laboratory data, the three variables of hematocrit, hemoglobin, and red blood count might show very high intercorrelations and might therefore be grouped together to form an index of erythematosity for making a simple diagnosis of anemia. Although this index might receive such mathematical approbations as a high value of Cronbach's alpha for its ingredients, a clinical user would immediately recognize that the three different variables are relatively synonymous. Most simple diagnoses of anemia could be made with any one of the three variables, not with all three.

The disparities between biologic and statistical coherence may create a major conflict of goals in the construction of composite indexes. Whenever possible, we would want to have good coherence in both bio- and -statistical attributes. If this double coherence cannot be obtained, a choice must be made about which type of coherence is preferable. Do we sacrifice biological plausibility in favor of statistical isometry, or do we retain isometry even when it does not make sense biologically? For example, we might use statistical isometry to form a cluster of objects all weighing **9-10 kg.** If the clustered objects, however, consist of young children, small dogs, and large fish, the cluster would have no distinct biological meaning.

Although the degree of preference for biologic vs. statistical coherence will vary from one circumstance to another, most scientists would insist that a direct conflict between the two should be resolved in favor of biologic coherence. A hypothesis based on biologic plausibility can always be rejected if not confirmed by statistical data; but statistical hypotheses are not intended to deal with issues in biology.[54] The ideas that emerge from statistical explorations of biologic data are meaningless unless shown to have biologic coherence. Despite the primacy of biology, however, the main point to be noted as we leave this section is that both types of coherence need careful consideration when indexes are constructed.

5.3.2. TRANSPARENCY OF CATEGORIES

The transparency of an output scale is a problem unique to aggregated composite indexes. *Transparency* refers to our ability to see through each output category to determine what it contains. To illustrate this idea, consider the Apgar score, which is an additive sum of the **0, 1,** or **2** ratings given to five different variables. If the total output score is **10** or **0,** we know exactly what component ratings it contains. For a score of **9** or **1,** we also have an excellent idea about the component ratings. If the total score is **5** or **6,** however, we know that the baby's condition is not splendid, but we do not know which clinical features are in trouble. An analogous problem arises if we use clustered categories, rather than scores, in the output scale. For example, the diagnostic cluster category of **acute rheumatic fever** does not indicate whether a patient has relatively benign arthritis without carditis, or severe carditis without arthritis.

This type of difficulty is unavoidable whenever multiple variables are combined into a single composite clinimetric index. The index may be satisfactory for offering a single output rating that summarizes the state of the included phenomena, but the particular components may become obscure enough to keep us from determining which ones are most responsible for the rating. If the output rating is our only concern, we have no real problem. Thus, an Apgar score of **5** creates no taxonomic difficulty if we merely want to classify the clinical condition of each of a series of newborn babies and if we then use the scores to get a statistical summary of the spectrum of newborns delivered on a particular perinatal service.

On the other hand, if we want to determine what proportion of the newborn babies have respiratory or cardiac abnormalities or if we want to estimate prognosis, choose treatment, or evaluate treatment for individual babies, the composite values of the Apgar score may be too imprecise for satisfactory usage. We might then need to disaggregate the total score into its individual elements or to develop some other index and scoring system for the additional clinical purposes.

Since the desire for a composite index and a transparent index may not be mutually compatible, the two goals must be carefully appraised when the index is constructed. In general, transparency is obtained by having the index contain a small number of variables and by rating and aggregating the variables in a simple manner. On the other hand, if we use only a few variables and a simple pattern of aggregation, we may not provide a satisfactory expression for the diverse component phenomena that we wanted to include in a composite index. The merit of a constructed index, therefore, may depend on the quality of the compromise achieved when priorities are assigned to the competing goals of transparency and adequate complexity.

5.4 Stipulation of Arrangement

The basic issues of reproducibility in clinimetric indexes usually occur, as noted in Chapter 3, in identifying the component variables and their demarcations. Since everything thereafter consists of combining the components, the main subsequent instructions should specify the mechanisms of combination and the output categories that emerge.

The combinatorial process takes place for axes as well as for output scales, because each axis (or subscale) is really a miniature output scale. As shown earlier in Figure 3.1, the process occurs sequentially as candidate variables are eliminated, as component variables are joined (when pertinent) to form axes (or subscales), as axes are combined to form an output scale, or as component variables are combined, without intermediate axes, to form the output scale directly. In each instance, we need to know the mechanism of combination and the identity of the ensuing categories.

5.4.1. FORMATION OF SCORES

If the combination consists of an arithmetical score, the stipulations are relatively simple. The arithmetical process is usually straightforward, readily shown with a mathematical formula, and easy to carry out. In most aggregated scores, the output is a simple sum of numerical ratings for the component elements or axes.

An interesting distinction in stipulation occurs when the values of the added ratings are expressed in global scales. The elemental global components will not have received demarcated stipulations, but their summated arrangement will be clearly specified. Thus, the categories will be well demarcated for the output scale, but not for its components.

5.4.2. PROBLEMS OF AMBIGUOUS AGGREGATION IN CLUSTERS

Unless suitable precautions are taken, ambiguous aggregations can readily occur when the output scale is expressed in Boolean clusters. The group of component categories can be arranged in many different ways, and the instructions must account for all possible arrangements. If all of them are not included, the output scale will have the ambiguities that were previously discussed in Section 5.1.3.

Problems of this type often arise if the component variables have ordinal ratings that are combined into an ordinal output scale. The table that shows the pattern of aggregation may seem quite clear, but may actually be grossly incomplete. For example, suppose an index has an ordinal output scale of **good, fair,** and **poor,** which is derived from three component variables, A, B, and C, each of which is also rated as **good, fair,** and **poor.** With three variables each having three possible ratings, we would expect the output scale to account for $27(=3^3)$ possible combinations. Nevertheless, the aggregation of components in the index may be presented as follows:

Rating in Output Scale	Rating for Categories of Component Variables		
	A	B	C
Good	Good	Good	Good
Fair	Fair	Fair	Fair
Poor	Poor	Poor	Poor

Instead of accounting for 27 possible arrangements of the components, this aggregation describes only the 3 patterns in which output ratings of **good, fair,** and **poor** are given to persons who have the same individual ratings in each component variable. We would not know how to rate a patient who is **good** in

A, **fair** in B, and **poor** in C, or who has any of the other 23 possible combinations.

Examples of this type of ambiguous aggregation can be seen in an index used to describe degree of activity in patients with rheumatoid arthritis.[33] Three graded ratings can be given to each of four variables: erythrocyte sedimentation rate, hemoglobin level, joint involvement, and systemic disturbance. The index scale is marked **inactive** if all four variables have the lowest rating, **moderately active** if all four variables have the middle rating, and **very active** if all four variables have the highest rating. No provision is made for other types of combinations where the constituent variables do not all have the same rating. This difficulty can be avoided in several ways. A pattern can be developed to account for all possibilities, the number of possibilities can be reduced by a hierarchical arrangement, or the constituent elements can be given numerical ratings that are added to form the output as a scored cluster.

Chapter 6

Indexes Requiring Active Collaboration by Patients

For most of the indexes that were actively constructed in Chapters 3, 4, and 5, the patient was relatively passive. The patient responded to questions or supplied other forms of information, but someone else designed and administered the index. All the main decisions in formulating ideas, choosing variables, demarcating scales, arranging combinations, and categorizing outputs were made either by the investigator who created the index or by the clinician who applied it.

Nevertheless, the patient is always an active collaborator in the total interchange that produces clinimetric data. When called upon merely to answer oral questions, the patient must be able to understand the questions and give suitable answers. When requested to answer a set of written questions, the patient must not only be able to understand the questions but must also be receptive enough to take the time and do the mental work involved in answering the questions. If asked to perform a physical rather than a mental task, the patient must be willing to exert suitable effort in responding to the physical challenges. In yet other situations, the patient can take a creatively active role in the focus of the index by expressing preferential choices about personal desires and satisfactions. If the patient's comprehension, receptivity, efforts, or preferences are not suitably recognized when the indexes are formulated and analyzed, the results can be distorted or misleading.

This chapter is concerned with the four types of patient collaboration that affect the structure and the results of clinimetric indexes. The collaborations occur when a patient supplies oral answers to questions asked by an examiner or interviewer; when a self-administered questionnaire requires suitable responses; when the patient is challenged to perform a physical task, such as exercising on a treadmill, walking up a flight of stairs, or working at a job; and when the multiple components of a complex attribute—such as physical function, social function, quality of life, or satisfaction with care— are rated for their desirability or importance.

6.1 Oral Responses

The histories taken by clinicians in daily practice are a classic example of clinimetric data supplied by patients as oral responses to questions. The activity is so familiar and so much an ingrained part of the ritual of routine patient care that most clinicians do not regard the work as a clinimetric exercise. Nevertheless, the information is regularly noted in medical records, and the data in the medical records are regularly reviewed, excerpted, coded, and analyzed to form the clinimetric indexes used in diverse types of medical research. In other investigations, the clinimetric information is obtained through a primary rather than a secondary process. The patient is directly interrogated by an interviewer who records the data immediately into special formats developed for the particular research that is being done.

Regardless of whether the patient's oral responses are entered in a routine medical record or a special research format, several important issues must be considered when the information is appraised as research data.

6.1.1. CONDITION OF THE PATIENT

An obvious first issue is the sensorial state of the patient. If the patient is mentally impaired—by disease, drugs, alcohol, or fatigue—the responses may be slightly inaccurate, grossly distorted, or bizarrely confabulated. An interviewer who fails to recognize the patient's mental state, however, may record all the erroneous information as though it were truth. An important early step in any interview, therefore, is to determine whether the patient's mental state and communication are good enough to be trusted.

A second important issue is to recognize the patient's possible motivation for providing incomplete or misleading answers. Many patients may be reluctant to confess holding beliefs or committing acts that are regarded as unfashionable, unpopular, immoral, or illegal. Unless this reluctance is recognized by the interviewer, the orthodox but erroneous responses submitted by the patient may also be accepted as accurate. Distortions of this type are particularly likely to occur when the quantity of intake or usage is described by smokers, alcoholics, or substance abusers, or when people with unconventional patterns of sex or personal relationships describe their activities. Other distortions may occur when patients with serious illness minimize their symptoms because of anxiety or denial, or when patients are unwilling to say things that might be potentially offensive to the clinician.

A third type of problem arises if patients exaggerate their physical infirmities or incapacities for reasons related to a pension, compensation, or an unresolved legal issue. All of these possibilities must be suitably considered before the patient's responses are accepted as being accurate and complete.

6.1.2. CONDITION OF THE INTERVIEWER

Since the patient's oral responses do not become data until recorded by the interviewer, the condition of the interviewer is another important factor. The interviewer's tactics in the interrogation can affect the patient's responses, and the interviewer's preconceptions about those responses can affect the way they are recorded.

Problems will often arise if clinicians have mistaken ideas about the correlation between symptoms and morphologic lesions; and many other beliefs, opinions, or hypotheses—as discussed elsewhere[38]—can lead to inaccurate or biased ascertainment of data. The main point to be noted now is that a potentially distorted interchange between patient and interviewer is an important issue that requires careful attention but that is often overlooked when clinimetric information is assembled.

6.2. Self-Administered Indexes

The possible adverse effects of an interviewer can be eliminated by eliminating the interviewer and letting the patient give direct written responses to a preplanned set of questions. This process, which is often called a self-administered questionnaire, is appealing because it saves time (at least for the interviewer) and it reduces the opportunity for interviewer-induced bias to occur in the answers. On the other hand, the absence of an interviewer also removes the flexibility with which questions can be phrased, elaborated, or followed up in an oral interrogation; and the absence of a personal interchange removes the opportunity to evaluate the condition of the responding patient. Furthermore, the acquired data become completely dependent on the quality and sequence of the stated questions and on the receptivity of the person who is asked to supply the answers.

Although many medical indexes describe events that occur during physical activity, the response to a set of questions requires mental activity and time. If no one is available to clarify any confusion produced either by the statements themselves or by the medium in which they are displayed, the respondent may give wrong answers. If the respondent is being asked to volunteer to do the work, the confusion may make the voluntary efforts stop before the questionnaire is completed. The efforts may also stop if the list of questions or the total procedure is so long that the respondent becomes bored, tired, disgruntled, or otherwise unwilling to continue.

Anyone who has taken a multiple-choice examination test is aware of the problems that can occur when a question (or the possible answer) is stated in an ambiguous manner. People who were previously unfamiliar with the operations of a computer terminal can readily recall the fear or anxiety they experienced unless the process was sufficiently user friendly. Recipients of an uninvited questionnaire in the mail will also recall the "short-fill phenomenon" that made them willing to respond to (and return) a few short statements, which required little time and effort, but unwilling to continue with a longer list, which often evoked a transfer of the questionnaire to the wastebasket.

For all these reasons, particular attention should be paid to verbal expressions, format of display, and total time duration of indexes that are to be self-administered. The verbal expressions should be reviewed for clarity and suitably tested in pilot studies to verify and improve clarity before the statements become formally employed. If the statements are displayed in a new or unfamiliar format, such as a computer terminal, the format itself requires scrutiny and pre-testing.

If the list of questions cannot be kept short, the investigators must consider the consequences of unanswered statements that come at the end of the list. For example, if the questionnaire contains a series of items for each of the sequence of four main topics A, B, C, and D, a fatigued or disgruntled recipient may offer no responses to any of the items for topic D occurring in the last part of the questionnaire. To avoid this type of problem in a long questionnaire, the investigator may arrange for items for all four topics to appear in a randomized sequence. This tactic will allow the early or pre-cessation responses to provide information for items in all four main topics, but the random presentation may also create confusion for the respondent, who wonders why the different topics have been jumbled together in an apparently illogical sequence of questions. Since no perfect approach is available, each situation of this type requires careful consideration in choosing a suitable sequence of statements, and the suitability of each sequence will usually depend on individual features of the contents, topics, and purpose of the questionnaire.

Many books have been written on the strategies and tactics used to construct self-administered questionnaires.[30,113,128] A particularly good text for clinical readers is Bennett and Ritchie's *Questionnaires in Medicine.*[7]

6.3. Task-Response Indexes

Many subjective sensations reported as apparently spontaneous symptoms actually involve responses to a task, and can be altered by altering the task. When pain occurs on exertion, inspiration, or movement, the patient can lower the level of the pain (or avoid it) by decreasing the effort used in the exertion, by breathing shallowly, or by moving slowly. In other instances, the results can be strikingly affected by the encouragement, goading, or other exhortations used to produce increased effort when a patient is asked to breathe deeply or walk vigorously during a particular test.

The responses to a task are commonly rated according to the magnitude of what is or is not accomplished. Thus, a forced vital capacity test is rated according to the volume of air moved, and a twelve-minute walking test, according to the distance covered during the walk. In other expressions of task magnitude, a patient may be rated as unable to work at a particular job or to climb two flights of stairs without discomfort.

For these ratings to be effective and clinimetrically valuable, several important features must receive suitable consideration in the interaction of the task and the patient. These features involve the magnitude of the task, the factors that affect the patient's effort in responding to the challenge, and the reasons for unsuccessful accomplishments.

6.3.1. MAGNITUDE OF TASK

For a task-response index to be applied effectively to different people, the magnitude of the task should be clearly understood and, if possible, standardized. For example, because different types of stairs have different lengths and degrees of inclination, a patient who cannot climb a flight of stairs in one location may readily do so in another. If a patient is unable to work at a job in the steel industry, what type of job produces the challenge: watchman, driver of a car, mover of heavy beams, or attendant at a furnace? In exercise-stress tests for coronary disease, the different mechanisms used for the exercise led to many inconsistent results until the various forms of portable steps, bicycle ergometers, and treadmill devices were brought into a standardized arrangement.

A separate problem in standardizing magnitude arises if the task produces a particular symptom, such as angina pectoris, dyspnea, or intermittent claudication. When a patient is recorded as having two-flight dyspnea, we do not know whether two flights of stairs are the *threshold* at which dyspnea first appears or the *maximum* that the patient can tolerate after the dyspnea begins. Since patients may vary greatly in their tolerance of symptoms and their willingness to continue a task after symptoms develop, the recorded magnitudes will be inconsistent if threshold and maximum values are not clearly distinguished.

6.3.2. COMPREHENSION OF TASK

The patient's comprehension of what must be done in a physical task is just as necessary as the understanding of instructions for a mental task. This comprehension is particularly important if the physical task involves an unfamiliar activity, such as the special maneuvers imposed in certain diagnostic procedures. For example, a patient who has never received laboratory tests of pulmonary function may not score well on the first set of tests because he is not sure of what is expected. On the second set of tests, after becoming a more experienced test taker, the patient may get better results. If the learning process or training effect is not appropriately discerned, the apparent improvement between the two sets of results may then be incorrectly attributed to the intervening therapy.

This phenomenon sometimes occurs in radiologic as well as clinimetric indexes. A patient receiving a chest X-ray for the first time may not yet have learned how to take and hold an adequately deep breath. On the second occasion, with deeper breathing, the heart may become more vertical, and the cardiothoracic ratio may seem smaller. The apparent decrease in cardiac size may then mistakenly be ascribed to the intervening treatment.

6.3.3. EXPOSURE TO TASK

In the exercise stress tests or pulmonary function tests conducted in clinical laboratories, the response is noted when the task is imposed directly upon the patient. In daily life, however, the patient decides what types of task to undertake. Consequently, a patient may not have been exposed to the challenge of certain tasks. For example, a patient may have had no recent opportunity to walk up two flights of stairs, to lift a heavy load, or to receive certain types of physical, social, or emotional stimuli. Unless the clinical observer is suitably attentive, the patient may be recorded as unable to perform certain tasks, although in fact the patient has not been recently challenged and does not know whether the tasks can actually be done.

This distinction is particularly important when the new ability to perform a previously unaccomplished task is used as an index of change. Encouraged after treatment to perform a certain task, the patient may do so successfully; the accomplishment may then be ascribed to the therapy unless we discover that the real change was from an initial state of unknown ability rather than known inability.

6.3.4. REASONS FOR NON-ACCOMPLISHMENT

When used as a clinical index, the non-accomplishment of a particular task is almost always attributed to the pathophysiologic consequences of whatever disease or condition is under study. Thus, if a patient with angina pectoris is not working, the inability to work is usually assumed to be a direct functional effect of the angina pectoris, which presumably occurs during the efforts required in the job. If the patient returns to work after medical or surgical treatment, the change is then ascribed to a pathophysiologic improvement produced by the treatment.

This assumption is frequently wrong because the patient may not have been working for many reasons other than the pathophysiologic effects of angina pectoris. In one instance, the patient may have lost his job or have been "laid off" for reasons unrelated to angina. In another instance, the patient may be unable to work because of a co-morbid disease, such as chronic emphysema or hepatic cirrhosis, rather than angina pectoris. The co-morbid ailment that sometimes impairs occupational capacity may be a psychiatric effect—such as depression—that was produced by the main disease or by some other cause. In yet another instance, the angina may have led to a pension or compensation plan that would vanish if the patient were to resume work. Finally, the patient may have stopped work for prophylactic reasons because of a physician's recommendation or because of his own fears that his cardiac condition might worsen.

In all of the foregoing situations, the task of work is not accomplished, but the patient was either non-exposed to the challenge of working or the non-accomplishment was due to other reasons. If the real reasons for non-accomplishment are not identified, a return to work after treatment of the principal condition will be incorrectly interpreted.

6.3.5. MAGNITUDE OF EFFORT

A different source of erroneous interpretations occurs when the magnitude of a task is increased while the concomitant magnitude of effort is disregarded. For example, the angina pectoris evoked by a particular task can almost always be prevented if the task is done with reduced vigor and effort. A patient who develops angina when climbing two flights of stairs at regular speed can easily become angina-free after (or without) treatment, by mounting the stairs much more slowly than before. If the reduction in effort is not noted, the new ability to climb two flights of stairs without angina may then be falsely credited to therapy.

One way of assessing effort is to measure the time required to perform a particular task. This technique has been used to assess the dexterity of elderly people, which was expressed as the total time required to complete a series of small manual tasks arranged on a special board.[156] The time needed for a task is not necessarily indicative, however, of the effort expended. For example, the distance walked in a fixed time was often dramatically increased when the patient was accompanied by a technician who offered encouragement or other inducement for extra effort while the walk was occurring.[77]

6.3.6. EFFECTS OF SUPPORT SYSTEM

In the example just cited, the patient's performance of a task was altered by concomitant attention and verbal exhortation. In many other circumstances beyond the clinical setting of a special test, the way that a patient copes with physical or emotional disabilities will be greatly affected by the available support system. This system consists of family, friends, or other persons who can offer physical aid, social assistance, emotional comfort, or other forms of help.

The role of the support system is frequently neglected when people are rated for disability in performing activities of daily living or other tasks. When two people with an apparently similar state of pathophysiologic impairment have different degrees of functional disability, the distinction is often regarded as an unpredictable, unexplained variation in human behavior. A simple inquiry about each person's associated support system, however, might readily indicate the reasons for the distinction. For example, of two similar people with the same type of bilateral amputations of the arms, one might be gainfully employed and the other be jobless. The difference could arise from the availability of someone at home to help when the prostheses are put on or taken off. Cooney et al.[19] have recently shown that despite severe impairment in activities of daily living, patients seldom needed placement in a nursing home if an adequate support system was available.

Consequently, for reasons discussed in this section and earlier in Section 6.3.5, the rating given for magnitude of task performance may not be an adequate account of the patient's ability (or disability) unless additional ratings are considered for magnitude of the patient's effort and support.

6.3.7. PROBLEMS OF INTERPRETATION

Although an index that describes response to a task cannot be properly interpreted merely from the particular crude rating or grade received by the patient, such crude ratings are pervasive in clinical literature today. They are constantly used, without suitable modifications or adaptations, in numerous indexes of cardiac and respiratory function, as well as in general indexes of functional capacity.

For satisfactory meaning and application, a task-response index must be suitably modified (or adjusted) to reflect the patient's motivation, effort, and support when responding to the task. Although intuitively sensed by many clinicians, the need for these modifications is seldom converted into formal action because the required information is usually regarded as being too complex or too "psychiatric" to be obtained without an extensive set of time-consuming questions. As noted in the foregoing discussion, however, the necessary information is easy to get if suitable efforts are made.

Relatively few additional questions are required, and they do not involve attention to any profoundly psychiatric topics. By finding the prophylactic, phobic, pathophysiologic, or other reasons for functional limitation, by determining whether an unaccomplished task was actually attempted, by asking about the vigor with which tasks are performed, and by noting the patient's motivation and social support, an investigator (or clinician) can readily acquire the data needed for the appropriate modifications. For example, a new clinical index of severity of dyspnea[118,149] for patients with chronic pulmonary disease contains provision for rating the magnitudes of both task and effort, and also for making appropriate distinctions (such as *not applicable*) when the dyspnea is caused by something other than lung disease.

Until appropriate modifications have been introduced and applied, many existing task-response indexes will not be fully suitable for the interpretations they usually receive.

6.4. Multi-Component Preferences

Among the main hazards of multi-component indexes are the risks of omitting, obscuring, or inadequately evaluating important information. After a brief review of the way those three problems can arise, the fourth part of this section contains a proposal of a "radical" solution for many of the problems: asking about the patient's preferences.

6.4.1. OMISSION OF COGENT ATTRIBUTES

In selecting the components of a composite index, the investigators may concentrate on variables that can readily be stipulated and rated. Consequently, important attributes that lack an existing system of formal expression may be overlooked or deliberately omitted. This type of difficulty is the source of many of the problems previously discussed throughout Section 6.3. The magnitude of a task is relatively easy to cite in quantitative terms, such as "climb two flights of stairs" or "walk 300 yards"; but such variables as the effort expended in doing the task, or the support system that may aid its performance, may be left out of the index because they are difficult to measure or because a suitable rating scale has not been established. The absence of suitable scales of expression is also responsible for the lack of attention in many prognostic indexes to such important clinical phenomena as severity of illness and severity of co-morbid disease.

These problems can easily be solved by recognizing the importance of the omitted attributes and by constructing suitable new indexes to identify them.

6.4.2. OBSCURITY OF IMPORTANT ATTRIBUTES

A different type of problem arises when an important variable is included in the composite index but is obscured by all the other things that are also included. The obscurity can arise from the surrounding subscales of a profile index or from the non-distinct expression produced by an aggregated index.

6.4.2.1. *Obscurity in Profile Indexes*

If a profile index contains ratings for many different subscales, the particular attribute that is the main focus of concern for a patient (or for a care giver) may be obscured among the many other subscale values. For example, suppose an index is expressed as a profile of ratings for subscales A, B, C, D, E, F, G, and H, and suppose subscale F is particularly important for the patient. If the initial rating is A2B3C4D1E5F4G3H2 and if the subsequent rating is A2B3C4D1E5F3G3H2, the improvement in subscale F may be of major value to the patient but may be lost or de-emphasized amid all the other ratings.

6.4.2.2. *Obscurity in Aggregated Indexes*

If the index just cited were expressed as an additive score rather than as a tandem profile, and if the score were obtained as a sum of the individual subscale ratings, the initial score for the cited patient would be 24 and the subsequent score would be 23. The reduction in score would be indicated by the change of one point, but the change would seem unimpressive because it is a proportional improvement of only about 4% (= 1/24). Nevertheless, from the patient's viewpoint, the main change, which has occurred only in the single subscale F, is a more impressive improvement of about 25% (= 1/4) in that scale.

Both types of obscuring problems just cited can be avoided if the important subscales are identified in advance, removed from their cohabitation with the other subscales, and used as separate indexes rather than as components of a larger combination.

6.4.3. INADEQUATE EVALUATIONS OF IMPORTANCE

In the problems just cited for multi-component indexes, important variables have been omitted or obscured. To regard these issues as problems, a mechanism is needed to make decisions about importance. In Section 4.3.2, we considered the judgmental and statistical strategies that can be used to evaluate importance when individual variables are candidates for inclusion in an index. After a variable has been chosen for inclusion, however, a different strategy is needed to decide about its relative importance with regard to all the other variables that have also been included in the composite index.

When this additional evaluation is applied, certain issues in the obscurity of component variables may turn out to be unimportant. For example, because a composite variable is intended to create a single summary expression for a complex phenomenon, the obscuring of individual components is an expected event. It does not create a problem, and is actually a desirable feature, if the index is being used exclusively as a summary statement. Thus, if we want to get an idea of the quantitative spectrum and average values of ratings for the condition of newborn babies in different hospitals, the Apgar score[5] would be an excellent index, even though the component ratings for individual variables such as heart rate, color, or tone are obscured in the total score. Similarly, if we wanted to compare the average degree of disability of groups of patients in nursing homes, we could effectively use the composite indexes developed by Barthel et al.[120] or by Katz et al.[98] even though the diverse component disabilities are not differentiated in the ratings of the output scale.

On the other hand, if the index contains descriptions of specific defects that are to be improved (or prevented) with clinical care, the impact on those defects cannot be specifically discerned unless the defects themselves are individually identified. For example, in the clinical scenario described in Section 6.4.2.1, the patient's total score might change from 24 to 23 after treatment aimed mainly at the condition cited in subscale B. Although the change of 24 to 23 in the total score might be regarded as improvement, a closer inspection of the component scores would show that no change had occurred in subscale B. The absence of the sought effect would not be noticed because the rating for subscale B had been obscured in the total rating summed from all the other subscales.

As a matter of pragmatic emphasis, therefore, certain variables may require specific identification when they are the direct focus of a therapeutic agent. For example, if an index contains a composite of ratings for pain, shortness of breath, peripheral edema, and anemia, an analgesic agent might be expected to affect the rating for pain, but not for the other variables. For such distinctions, the composite index might be "decomposed" into a separate subscale rating for pain, which would then become the focus of attention in evaluating the analgesic agent.

A different issue arises, however, when a more general form of therapy— such as an anti-inflammatory agent or rehabilitation procedure—can affect several different variables rather than just one. For example, a patient with severe rheumatoid arthritis may have difficulties in fine hand movements, in dressing, in ambulation, and in occupational capacity. When such a patient is treated with anti-inflammatory agents or with physical therapy, not all these disabilities may be susceptible to improvement. Similarly, a patient who is incapacitated in mobility, basic hygiene, excretory continence, and other activities of daily living may not be immediately capable of improvement in all the disabilities. What should be emphasized when multiple disabilities are treated, and how should the choice be made?

If we make the choice with a mathematical form of analysis, as discussed in Section 4.3.2, the decision depends on a statistical algorithm that can be greatly affected by arbitrary mathematical ideas in the algorithm and by the numbers of cases contained in the processed data. If the decision is made using clinical judgment, the choice may depend upon the personal values and beliefs of the clinician making the judgment. Regardless of how well those decisions are made, they may be basically inadequate if they do not allow relative importance to be chosen by the person for whom each decision is most cogent.

6.4.4. COGENT DECISIONS AND PERSONAL PREFERENCES

Suppose a patient with mild nonincapacitating congestive heart failure can be treated in a way that will relieve either dyspnea or peripheral edema but not both. Who should choose the single target to be relieved? Suppose a medical student who is receiving low grades in Subject A and Subject B can receive tutorial help in only one of them. Who picks the subject that will be helped?

Questions of this type are not always easy to answer because the choices may not always be evenly divided. One of the choices may sometimes be mandated or favored by external factors, not stated in the text of the questions, that strongly affect the decision. For example, if the patient with congestive heart failure has chronic lung disease and the year is at the height of the "flu" season, the attempt to reduce dyspnea may seem more important than a reduction of peripheral edema. Similarly, if the medical student wants to be a surgeon, tutorial help in surgery may seem more important than help in psychiatry.

On the other hand, if all other factors are indeed equal, a strong case can be made for letting the choice of personal focus or preference be made by the person for whom the decision is most important. Thus, if an index is being used to determine or emphasize activities performed by the staff at a nursing home, the choice should depend upon goals selected by the staff. On the other hand, if the index expresses the desires of a patient or a patient's family, the choice should be made by him, her, or them.

Despite the obvious rationale for letting choices of this type be made by the most cogently affected people, the strategy has not been commonly used in medical care. In particular the strategy has not been applied as a relatively simple method for choosing the focal emphasis of care according to selections made by the patients or other non-clinical people (such as family members) who are most intimately affected by the care. Nevertheless, one patient with severe problems in use of extremities may not be distressed by trouble in walking as long as she can use her hands for fine movements. Another patient may have the reverse preference. A third patient may not care about either walking or fine hand movements as long as she can continue to think and express her thoughts vigorously. Unless these preferences are discerned, both the treatment and its evaluation may be aimed at the wrong thing.

The importance of patients' preferences is now well recognized in activities such as quantitative decision analysis,[154] where "utility values" must be established for the different types of outcome events that might occur after certain clinical decisions. To determine these utility values, investigators have developed elaborate strategies for attempting to elicit patient preferences and to convert those preferences into the quantitative units that can be used in the mathematical models of the decision-analysis procedure. These elaborate strategies are often not needed if the clinimetric index allows a patient's preferences to be expressed simply and directly, without recourse to quantitative transformations.

It is difficult to determine why the importance of patients' preferences has been so ignored in most indexes of general function or quality of life. Except for a recent effort by Pincus et al.[132] to assess "patient satisfaction in activities of daily living," almost no attempts have been made to ask patients directly what they want or would like to have. The various weights of importance for the diverse variables contained in health status indexes are usually assigned by a mathematical model or the judgmental values of a clinical observer or investigator, but the preferences of the patient are seldom solicited and incorporated into the indexes. Perhaps the main reason for this neglect is the fear that different preferences might lead to non-standard indexes. This fear can promptly be eliminated, however, if we decide on a standard scale for measuring improvement, but let the patient's preference govern the choice of the particular variable in which the improvement will be measured.

The expression of patients' preferences is valuable not only in health status indexes but also in indexes that deal with any form of satisfaction. For example, suppose an index is being developed to cite a patient's satisfaction with clinical care. We might ask the patient to rate such attributes as the clinician's personality, courtesy, availability, communication, and procedural skills (in such jobs as drawing blood).[121] An overall combination of these ratings will not be effective, however, unless we determine how relatively important those attributes are to the patient. If the patient cares little about personality but a great deal about communication, a doctor who is rated low in personality but high in communication should receive a better summary rating for that patient than a doctor who is rated high in personality but low in communication.

Until these distinctions in patients' preferences and desires are better managed, many existing multi-component indexes will continue to be unsuitable for the job they are assigned to do in expressing states of general function, satisfaction, or quality of life.

Chapter 7

Global Indexes and Scales

Two main principles are usually required in a scientific process of measurement: standardized content and standardized scale. For example, if we wanted to measure serum glucose, we would first need a standardized method that correctly identifies glucose as the content of the measurement. We would then need a standardized scale that indicates the magnitude of the glucose.

In clinimetric procedures, the standardization of content occurs via an explicit specification of the variables included in the index. The standardization of scale occurs with stipulated directions for demarcating each of the ratings in the output scale. When multiple variables are included in a composite index, the directions should indicate how to demarcate the ratings of the scale for each component variable, and also how to combine those ratings to form the output scale of the composite index.

These two principles are not fulfilled when an index is expressed in an output scale that has no operational demarcations for its ratings. The ratings in the scale can be expressed in visual analog, ordinal, binary, or nominal format; but the different categories or ratings are not demarcated with stipulated criteria. The selections are made by individual raters as an act of feeling, perception, opinion, or belief, using whatever personal standards seem appropriate for the task.

For example, an index for *improvement after treatment* might be expressed in a scale with two binary categories, such as **not improved** and **improved;** or the scale might have an ordinal array of categories, such as **much worse, slightly worse, same, slightly improved, greatly improved.** The scale might also be presented in visual analog form:

|———————————————————————————————————————|

Substantially   *Completely*
  Worse   *Improved*

With any one of these binary, ordinal, or visual analog scales, patients could offer a simple direct indication of their improvement after treatment, and an investigator could use the data immediately in whatever study is being done. On the other hand, in the absence of criteria for the selected choices, we would not know what the patients were actually thinking about as manifestations of improvement, or precisely what magnitudes of change had led to the individual ratings.

7.1. Nomenclature and Structure of Global Indexes

There is no standard name for indexes that lack a demarcated scale. The term *global* is well accepted and often used when the content of the index refers to a broad overview of a complex phenomenon, such as *improvement after treatment* or *general health status.* Such indexes do not have criteria to identify either the component variables or the choice of output ratings that were used in the overview. We would not know what things the patient included or excluded in making decisions about improvement or health, and why those things received high or low ratings.

In other indexes that do not have demarcated ratings, the content may be identified (usually in the title) as a reasonably specific clinical entity, such as *severity of dyspnea, severity of chest pain,* or *degree of cardiac enlargement.* Some investigators will call such indexes *uncalibrated* or *undemarcated* and will prefer to save *global* as a label for an index with a larger scope of unstipulated content. Nevertheless, although *severity of dyspnea* seems more specific than *improvement after treatment,* we still would not know what things the patient was thinking about in rating the severity of dyspnea.

An argument might be offered that even a clearly specified content, such as *severity of chest pain,* is not really well specified. We do not know whether the rating of severity depends on the intensity, duration, quality, or location of the pain, and whether the rating was affected by the patient's psychic status. A counter-argument might then be offered that the target phenomenon has been reasonably well specified because we know (or can assume) that it is chest pain rather than something else. In a global index for *improvement after treatment,* we have very little idea of what phenomena have been included or how they have been weighted and combined.

To avoid invidious decisions about scope or specification of content, the word *global* will be used here for indexes that do not have a specifically demarcated scale for the output ratings. In most instances, the indexes refer to a broad global entity whose exact contents are unidentified, but sometimes the entity will seem more specific. In either instance—with either a broad or a narrow focus in content—we will not know exactly what has been observed and how it has been evaluated, because the output scale is not accompanied by operational criteria for demarcating the ratings. Since globality of content and demarcation need not be distinguished for the ensuing discussion, the exact nomenclature is relatively unimportant as long as the idea is clear.

7.2. **Advantages and Disadvantages of Global Indexes**

Global indexes have major advantages and disadvantages. They are simple, direct, easy to construct, and easy to use; but the data come from unstandardized demarcations and often from unspecified components. Because of the advantages, global indexes are constantly used in clinical communication to describe patients' conditions and reactions. Because of the disadvantages, global indexes do not have the reproducibility demanded of scientific data. In the absence of specifications for rating a patient's condition as **4+ sick,** a response to treatment as **excellent,** or satisfaction with care as **high,** the results cannot be replicated. An outside observer cannot determine exactly what was examined, what was thought about it, and what components were combined to form the global rating.

Global indexes dramatically illustrate the conflict that often arises in the competing scientific goals of clinical measurement. The indexes have almost all the virtues of sensibility, but few of the merits of standardization. In sensibility, we need not worry about whether a global index gives a suitable description of a particular phenomenon, because the rating is directly aimed at the phenomenon. It has not been altered or misrepresented by selected variables that provide objective, dimensional, standardized data aimed tangentially or at some other phenomenon. A global index for severity of chest pain describes severity of chest pain, not the measurements of waves in an electrocardiogram. A global index for clinical severity of dyspnea describes clinical severity of dyspnea, not a laboratory measurement of forced expiratory volume.

Nevertheless, without knowing what the patients (or clinicians) have in mind when they rate the severity of chest pain or dyspnea, we cannot regard the information as having the reproducible consistency that is a sine qua non of hard scientific data. In the absence of reproducible consistency, the information provided by global indexes is often disdained as soft, and the important human phenomena described by the indexes are often omitted from scientific analysis. The hard data used in the research may then yield results that are scientifically respectable but clinically defective.

A prime scientific challenge in clinimetrics today is to construct indexes that can achieve a satisfactory compromise among several competing goals: the consistency needed for general science, the suitability needed for clinical science, and the simplicity needed for pragmatic clinical usage.

7.3. **Historical Development of Global Scales in Medicine**

The origins of global medical scales are difficult to determine. The **1+, 2+,..., 4+** system that is constantly used in medical communication today was probably imported into clinical work from its prior use to express the results of laboratory tests. The "plus" system was used at least as early as 1911 in Craig's scale[22] of **–, +–, +, ++** to record the results of the Wasserman serologic test for syphilis. In 1917, Craig[23] wrote that other laboratories were reporting Wasserman test results using the scale of **+, ++, +++, ++++**. As the Wasserman test became used and discussed throughout the world of medicine, the **1+,..., 4+** scale was probably carried over into clinical work to grade the relative magnitude of such entities as symptoms and clinical conditions that could not be cited in dimensional expressions.

While the plus system was being diffused into clinical work, psychosocial scientists were following a parallel but slightly different approach. Although ordinal scales were being used, according to Boring,[12] "at the turn of the century," the graphic rating scale described earlier in Section 3.1.2 seems to have been first proposed by Hayes and Patterson[82] in 1921 as a method of rating occupational performance. In a review two years later, Freyd[67] discussed the use of graphic rating scales but also described a tactic that resembles a visual analog scale. Freyd implied that the visual analog scale had been developed before the graphic rating scale, but gave no reference for the statement.

Visual analog scales first seem to have been applied for medical phenomena in 1964, when Clarke and Spear[15] reported that such scales were both sensitive and reliable for citing patients' self-rating of well-being. Writing in the *Proceedings of the Royal Society of Medicine* a few years later in 1969, Aitken[2] recommended that visual analog scales be used for the measurement of feelings. Although these two publications seemed to offer the pioneering exhortations, visual analog scales remained relatively neglected in clinical research until Huskisson et al.[89] in 1974 demonstrated the effectiveness of the scales for measuring pain in arthritic patients.

Until Huskisson's work brought the visual analog scale into clinical prominence, pain was being rated in an alternative manner, with ordinal categories. An adjectival scale for pain—using the categories **nil, slight, moderate, severe,** and **agony**—was proposed in the United Kingdom by

Keele[99] in 1948. In 1949, Hewer et al.[83] assigned the numerical values of **0, 1, 2, 3,** and **4** to the Keele scale to simplify the recording of the verbal descriptions. An analogous set of ordinal categories, expressed in the same verbal terms (except for *agony*) as the Keele scale, was developed independently in the United States by Houde[85] in 1951 and was used in 1954 in a study done by the National Academy of Science,[85] but the first formal account[84] of the Houde scale did not appear until 1960.

Houde later converted his verbal categories to numerical ratings, which were then used to measure the course of pain relief as a Sum of Pain Intensity Differences at various time points. The tactic was christened as the SPID index by Forrest et al.[66] in 1963, when they also introduced a separate four-category transition scale for expressing pain relief directly rather than as an incremental difference in successive single-state ratings. In 1970, Huskisson et al.[88] expanded the scope of the ratings by introducing a nine-category transition scale for assessing pain relief.

During the past 15 years, various investigators have compared visual analog scales vs. categorical scales in the assessment of pain and other symptoms. The results have not shown a clear superiority for either of the two sets of approaches. In some circumstances[93,127,142,148] the visual analog scales seemed better than categorical scales, but in other circumstances[32,79,114] the categorical scales were preferred. Relatively few studies have been done to compare transition scales vs. repeated use of single-state scales in the measurement of change. In two recent reports, transition scales seemed particularly effective.[118,141]

The best usage of the different formats for global scales remains to be determined in future research. As with other types of indexes, the optimal formats will probably vary according to the purpose of each index and the framework and setting in which it is used.

7.4. **Internal (Within-Person) Standardization**

Despite the apparent imprecision of a scale that has no operational demarcations, global ratings can be used in a reasonably standard manner when repeatedly applied by the same person. Although different people will obviously use different criteria when they rate the severity of their own chest pain on a global scale of **0, 1, 2, 3,** or **4,** or on a visual analog line, each person will presumably use the same individual criteria when he rates his own pain. The scale can therefore be reasonably consistent when used repeatedly to show transitions in the state of each patient.

For example, two patients who give their pain the ratings of **4, 3,** and **1** on three successive occasions can be properly regarded as having achieved substantial improvement in the sequential response, even if they employed different concepts for their own individual single-state ratings of severity of pain. This attribute of global indexes makes them particularly valuable for denoting changes in state. Although the individual ratings are not standardized among the individual patients, they will be reasonably well standardized within the same patient.

7.5. External (Among-Persons) Standardization

When used to denote a single state, the ratings of a global index will not be standardized for the different people who use it. On the other hand, if the different people are all rated by the same person, and if that person is reasonably consistent, the ratings may be standardized despite the absence of demarcational criteria. For example, if the same clinician applies the same global index to rate severity of chest pain or severity of illness for each member of a group of patients, the results might be well standardized. Conversely, if the index is self-administered and the patients give themselves their own ratings, the likelihood of standardization is small.

This problem is not unique in rating severity of pain, severity of illness, or other phenomena with indexes that seem obviously global. The same problem occurs whenever an index contains subjective ratings expressed in a scale whose demarcations have not been explicitly identified and tested. For example, substantial inconsistencies and lack of standardization are regularly found within the same observer and among different observers when histopathologists are studied for variability in identifying the cell types of lung cancer,[42] when radiologists decide whether a plain chest film shows pulmonary embolism,[74] and when coronary arteriographers rate the status of coronary vasculature.[27] Although the information supplied by these observers is ordinarily accepted as scientific data, the ratings are often given with scales that are essentially global because the operational demarcations are either not fully specified or not applied in a standardized manner.

7.6. Standardization of Transitions

Although a global index may not be standardized when different people rate a single state, the ratings may be reasonably well standardized, both internally and externally, for ratings of change. Within the same person, as noted earlier, the same operational criteria will presumably be used to produce a sequence of ratings such as **4, 3,** and **1.** Some other person, with a sequence of **3, 1,** and **0** may have used different criteria for the individual ratings, but if we decide to rate the sequence as **substantially improved** for each person, the transition rating can be standardized because its component features (such as a sequence of **4-3-1** or **3-1-0**) show a consistent trend and have been overtly specified.

A single-state global index can thus be reasonably well standardized when used repeatedly to show changes, particularly if the focal content of the indexes is well standardized. If the index refers to a specific pain or discomfort (rather than to a more general phenomenon, such as health status), the individual raters will presumably be consistent in their individual ratings, the change or trend shown in the individual ratings can be cited in appropriate patterns, and the patterns can then be used as standardized ratings.

A similar type of standardization can be achieved if the change is expressed globally in a direct transition scale such as **−2, −1, 0, +1, +2,** or **worse, same, better.** Although individual raters may have different criteria for such *single*-state ratings as **mild** and **severe,** the raters are much more likely to use similar criteria when they indicate *transition* ratings, such as **better** or **worse.**

This distinction illustrates another advantage of global scales. A collection of single-state global ratings for a group of people may be too unstandardized for the spectrum of results to be collected and summarized as a "legitimate" variable, but a collection of transition ratings may be reasonably well standardized within and among the individual members of the group. This distinction is probably the reason global transition scales have been so clinically popular and well accepted for expressing responses to therapy, or other changes in clinical course.

7.7. **Problems in Bias and Standardization**

Because everything is so subjective, global ratings can be affected by biases arising in any one (or more) of three different levels of the observational process: perception, reporting, and repeat observations. At the perceptual level, bias can affect the way in which a person perceives a sensation (such as pain) and forms a response. At the reporting level, bias can alter the category of the rating in which the response is reported. At the repeat observation level, bias may alter the subsequent rating that is chosen after an initial rating.

Several methods can be used in attempts to prevent these problems. The most obvious and best known procedure is the double-blind technique for evaluating medication. In this technique, the identity of the medication is hidden from both the patient and the doctor so that neither person will have expectations that can affect perceptions and responses. An analogous procedure can be used to produce a "blind" observer when the complete observational process can be accomplished by only one person, such as a radiologist or pathologist, who need not see the patient directly and who can be denied any information that might prejudice the process.

The same type of blinding can be maintained to avoid bias when the basic observations are converted into reported data. As an additional precaution to help standardization, however, the scale used for the reports may be displayed so that it confronts each reporter in the same way when a report is prepared. Thus, rather than being offered in "open" or "fill-in-the-blank" response, the observer may be asked to check or circle a choice among a specified group of categories or to mark a location on a labeled visual analog scale.

A different type of problem arises when the observer is asked to repeat a single-state rating, which will be compared with the previous rating for calculating an increment, ratio, or some other distinction that denotes a change in state. Arguments can be offered both for and against the policy of letting the observer see the previous rating when the new one is made.[78] The argument in favor of hiding the previous rating is that it may bias the observer's current response. The argument for letting the observer see the previous rating is that it will help standardize, i.e., increase the consistency of, the second response. Thus, a patient who feels slightly improved, but who does not remember the exact location of his previous mark on the single-state visual analog scale, may make a blind response that does not suitably indicate the slight improvement. Regardless of which argument seems more persuasive, the problem can be avoided by using a separate transition scale, rather than a repetition of the same single-state scale, for repeated responses. With a transition scale, the observer can directly record the slight improvement or other change in state, without having to remember or review the previously recorded response.

7.8. Graphic Aids to Comprehension

A different type of challenge in global scales is to ensure that the users understand what is being requested. The observer's comprehension of the basic question is always an important issue in any index, regardless of the detailed quality of the instructions and scale that are provided for the answer. Because a global scale is not accompanied by criteria for demarcating the ratings, however, the rater may have an extra problem in understanding how to use the scale. For example, elderly people with chronic disease were found in one study[107] to have been confused by the challenge of marking a visual analog scale. In other circumstances, someone who is accustomed to expressing ratings in verbal categories, such as **poor, fair, good, excellent,** may have trouble transposing the ratings to numerical grades such as **1, 2, 3,** and **4.** Someone who is accustomed to numerical ratings that have **10** as the top grade may be uncomfortable with a rating system in which the peak value is **5, 6,** or **7.** Other issues, as discussed in Section 5.2 and elsewhere,[14,124] involve the number of categories to be included in a rating scale, the observer's ability to discriminate among the categories, and the ability of the categories to discriminate among the basic phenomena to be distinguished.

One interesting recent contribution has been the use of pictures or other graphic displays to portray ratings that are better seen visually than described verbally. For example, in studying maternal psychological determinants of infant obesity, Kramer et al.[106] developed four drawings of nine-month-old children with body habitus ranging from lean to chubby. The scale of portraits for girls is shown in Figure 7.1. When mothers were asked to rank the four drawings in order of preference for the ideal body habitus they wanted for their new baby, the results showed striking correlations with the mother's age, socioeconomic status, and subsequent patterns in feeding the children. The investigators have thus shown that a set of well-chosen pictures can sometimes replace hundreds of words as demarcational criteria for categories of a scale.

7.9. Problems in Stipulation of Components

Although the absence of demarcated standardization will always be a scientific handicap when global output scales are used as instruments of measurement, the most basic problem occurs in standardizing the content of the variables included in an entirely global index. When a patient is rated as **severely ill, 4+ sick,** or **95** on a 100-mm visual analog scale of *illness severity,* we have no idea of exactly what is wrong or what to do about it. Similarly, when response to therapy is given a rating of **good,** did the response occur because the symptoms themselves were better, because the patient was less anxious about them, or because the patient's attention to the illness was distracted by other events?

If we want to know what is really happening, a global index will not stipulate the necessary components of the fundamental observations. This defect may seem to be an overwhelming scientific flaw of global indexes— until we recall that the same flaw occurs in almost every index constructed as a composite of multiple demarcated components. Thus, although the Apgar score has a well-demarcated output scale, with component variables that are well identified and well demarcated in their own elemental scales, the identity of the component parts is blurred when the score is expressed in its composite output. We would not know exactly what was wrong if a baby had an Apgar score of **5,** and we would not know the specific thing or things that had improved if the score changed from **5** to **7.** Similarly, the *wind-chill factor* is a composite index constructed of data that have impeccable scientific creden-

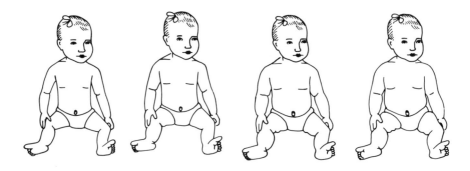

Figure 7.1. *Drawings of female infants used by Kramer et al. for maternal perceptions of Ideal Body Habitus. (Scale ranges from 1 = leanest, at far left, to 4 = most obese, at far right.)*

Source: M. S. Kramer, R. G. Barr, D. G. Leduc, C. Boisjoly, and I. B. Pless, "Maternal Psychological Determinants of Infant Obesity: Development and Testing of Two New Instruments," *J. Chron. Dis.* 1983;36:329–35.

tials, but we do not know whether a wind-chill factor of **−20** represents mainly wind, mainly chill, or roughly equal parts of both.

The demand for precise identification is an obvious necessity of science—but the demand is appropriate only if it matches the particular goal of the scientific activity. When we form a composite index or a global scale for a complex phenomenon, the scientific goal is to get an overall appraisal of the total phenomenon, not to preserve the identity of each component. If we want to know about the components, we would use or review separate indexes for the components. Thus, if we want to determine what is wrong with a baby whose Apgar Score is **5,** we would check the separate scales used for each of the Apgar components. We would also check those same separate scales to see which ones had changed when the score went from **5** to **7.** Similarly, if we wanted to know the sources of a wind-chill factor of **−20,** we would examine the separate component values for wind and for temperature. Analogously, if we want to know the exact features that are involved when severity of illness is expressed in a global rating of **4+ sick** or **95,** we cannot use the global rating itself. Instead, we would have to prepare and inspect individual ratings for each of the various features.

7.10 **Conflicts in Choice of Scientific Goals**

Although often highly desirable for many scientific activities, the goal of describing a complex phenomenon in a single composite index may be incompatible with the simultaneous goal of preserving the identity of the individual components. If we want to attain both goals, we can do so by using separate indexes for the whole and for the parts; but the important scientific contributions of composite indexes (and global scales) will not be fairly evaluated if they are expected to hit the wrong target.

As discussed later in Chapter 10, global indexes are particularly valuable as the best way to describe complex phenomena that may not be suitably and simply expressed if observations of the phenomena are formally decomposed into component parts and then formally reconstituted into a clearly demarcated scale. The desirable consistency achieved with a formal decomposition-reconstruction process may involve an unacceptably high loss of suitability and simplicity. As noted in this chapter, global indexes are not as inconsistent as they seem to be on superficial appraisal; and certain types of standardization can readily be expected or attained when the indexes are used. Other improvements in standardization can also be achieved, without losing the advantage of global simplicity, if creative attention is given to the format and display of the global scale.

A fundamental problem that may impede creative attention to global indexes, however, is the belief that they are not worth improving because they are inherently unscientific. They do not seem to fulfill the basic scientific requirements for standardized content and standardized scale. This scientific dismissal of global indexes often occurs, however, because the other scientific virtues of the indexes are either forgotten or undervalued when priorities are chosen among several competing scientific goals.

The competition of goals is a particularly crucial basic scientific issue in clinimetrics. The choice and emphasis of scientific goals for an index, and the policies adopted in pursuing those goals, will affect every aspect of the strategy with which an index is constructed and evaluated.

A choice among reasonable but competing goals is not a unique problem in clinimetrics. The same type of problem also occurs in other clinical activities. In plans for randomized clinical trials, the design and analysis of a trial will be different (and often disputed) when a choice is made between a *pragmatic* and a *fastidious* goal.[54] The decisions made in medical ethics will be different (and often disputed) when a choice is made between *samaritan* and *societal* goals.[54] In clinimetric activities, an analogous conflict may arise when both "standardization" and "sensibility" are sought as scientific goals. Although both goals may be equally important and desirable, a single index may effectively be able to achieve one or the other, but not both. The designers of the index will then have to decide which goal should receive priority.

This conflict is seldom openly recognized when clinicians collaborate with statistical and psychosocial consultants in constructing clinimetric indexes. The consultants work with a well-established set of policies that provide a distinctive theory for their work. The theory contains principles and strategy for achieving the summarization, variance reduction, "reliability," "validity," and other attributes that aim at standardization as a prime scientific goal in forming indexes. This goal is usually accepted without further discussion, and the possible conflict with other goals is not considered because clinicians have no analogous theory with which to state the alternative goals of "sensibility."

Clinicians have generally given so little attention to clinimetric strategy that an analogous theory, with distinctive policies and procedures, has not been developed for citing sensibility as an important additional primary scientific goal. The idea of theory may even seem strange when applied to issues in clinical measurement. Through various educational exposures and background in science, clinicians might readily be able to outline the theory or principles needed for satisfactory measurement of laboratory data, but similar ideas have not been developed for clinimetric activities. The process of history taking, physical examination, and clinical reasoning is taught and used for its role in making pathophysiologic or clinical decisions, but not as an exercise in scientific measurement. The scientific theory used in clinical work refers to paradigmatic concepts of etiologic agents, pathophysiologic mechanisms, and therapeutic or prophylactic interventions, but not to any paradigms in clinical forms of measurement. Consequently, when collaborating with statistical or psychosocial consultants, clinicians are usually unaware of the existence of theory in measurement, and may not know that the consultant works with a particular theory having a particular goal.

Furthermore, without a formal theory of their own, clinicians either may not recognize that alternative goals exist or may not be able to express them articulately. The clinician's silence is usually abetted by the knowledge that standardization has always been a prime goal of scientific data, by the consultant's clear sense of direction, and by the frequent confusion or awe produced by the concomitant mathematical activities. Consequently, standardization may become the only goal that is identified, or the goal that receives priority in all decisions when an index is formulated. The result is often highly successful, but it also often fails because neither the clinicians nor the consultants recognized that the wrong goals were being emphasized.

To help avoid some of these problems, the next three chapters are devoted to the goals and policies that constitute the underlying theory for the practice conducted when statisticians, psychosocial scientists, and clinicians formulate indexes. Chapters 8 and 9 are concerned with statistical and psychosocial approaches to standardization. Chapter 10 describes the principles of clinical approaches to sensibility. An awareness of the similarities and of certain important differences in those underlying approaches can advance the artful science of clinimetric indexes by enabling the clinicians and the consultants to understand more about one another's work. This increased understanding can then help improve the quality of communication and fertility of products in the interdisciplinary collaboration.

Chapter 8

The Goals of Statistical Methods

Although the creators of a process of measurement always want it to do a good job, the decision about what constitutes a "good job" depends on the choice of goals. The goals are usually set according to beliefs about what is necessary or desirable when a particular index is constructed and tested. For example, someone who wants scientific measurements to be expressed in dimensional scales will be dissatisfied with any scales that are non-dimensional. A devout believer in demonstrations of accuracy may be scientifically discontent with any indexes that have not been tested for accuracy—even if the test is impossible because a suitable reference standard does not exist.

These and many other beliefs about the desirable goals of a measurement process are not always overtly cited when an index is developed, but they affect almost every phase of the development. At each step in the process, different options are chosen for policies that reflect the underlying beliefs. Such options are exercised when the creator of an index chooses its focus and component observations; decides to form it as an arithmetical score rather than as a cluster; uses 2, 3, 7, or 24 categories in the output scale; transforms or retains the basic expressions of observed data; assigns weights and aggregations with judgmental rather than mathematical strategies; arranges for the index to receive a planned field test; and establishes standards for interpreting the results of the test.

Despite their profound impact on the choice of options, the basic beliefs about desirable goals are seldom formally specified. Consequently, the different beliefs held by different professional groups are seldom formally recognized. In the absence of such recognition, members of these groups—working alone or in collaboration—may seem to have similar objectives in creating an index, but the options used to approach the objectives may differ substantially. This type of problem often arises when clinicians collaborate with statistical or psychosocial consultants. The collaborators may seem to seek the same thing while pursuing it with distinctively different basic goals and policies that lead to major differences in the results.

If the result is successful, everyone may be happy; but if things do not go well, the collaborators may not discern the underlying problems—arising from conflicting goals and policies—that led to the difficulties. In some instances, the collaborators may be particularly puzzled or distressed when a result that seems excellent as an act of biometry or psychosocial measurement turns out to be inadequate as an act of clinimetrics.

The purpose of this chapter, and of the two that follow it, is to improve the quality of the interdisciplinary collaboration by bringing open recognition to the different basic goals and policies used when indexes are created by statistical, psychosocial, and clinical investigators. In this chapter, the focus is on differences in statistical and clinical approaches. Chapters 9 and 10 contain analogous attention to differences in psychosocial and clinical activities.

8.1. Distinctions in Statistical and Clinical Goals

An example of contrasting professional viewpoints was noted in Section 5.3 as the distinction between clinical and statistical ideas about coherence. Statistically, a series of different items would be grouped together if the items have certain quantitative similarities or isometry. Clinically, the items are grouped together on a qualitative basis if their combination is justified by a suitable biologic concept. The items may be manifestations of the same disease or pathophysiologic derangement; they may be different etiologic agents (or risk factors) for a disease; they may be prognostic factors that predict a poor outcome—but the link that holds them together is a specific idea that has the plausibility of biologic logic.

In statistical goals, these ad hoc acts of judgmental reasoning are deliberately excluded from consideration. The statistical approaches call for decisions that are made with mathematical models, having their own intrinsic logic and rationale, that will always produce a consistent and correct result within the framework of that model. The idea is to have a model that will function effectively within its own mechanism of operation, regardless of what types of data are entered into the model. For example, when we use a formula such as $\overline{X} = \Sigma X_i / N$ for a mean, or $s = \sqrt{\Sigma(X_i - \overline{X})^2/(n - 1)}$ for a standard deviation, the mathematical model will be applicable regardless of what biologic attribute is considered as the variable X. If the mathematical model happens to produce either a peculiar biologic result, such as a statement that the average family has 2.3 children, or a misleading result, such as mean income values that are distorted by people who are extremely wealthy "outlyers," the inappropriateness of the result must be appraised with clinical rather than mathematical reasoning.

The mathematical models used in clinimetric activities for two different statistical purposes—description and inference—will be briefly discussed in the next two sections.

8.1.1. DESCRIPTIVE STATISTICS

The mathematical models of descriptive statistics can produce indexes that are statistical, clinical, or both. The most common statistical expressions in clinical literature are an "index of central tendency," such as a mean, median, or proportion, and an "index of dispersion," such as a standard deviation or inner-percentile range. These statistical expressions are used to summarize the spectrum of a particular group of univariate data. The central index and index of dispersion (or spread), for example, would give the summary values for weight, for blood pressure, for age, and for gender in a group of people. The individual summaries could then be compared in two or more groups of people.

Another type of statistical index offers a mathematical description of the association between two or more variables. Thus, the relationship between weight and blood pressure, or among age, height, weight, and blood pressure, could be expressed with regression coefficients and correlation coefficients. These statistical indexes of association often have a prominent role in clinimetric work because the magnitude and variance of the coefficients can be a prime focus of consideration in decisions about the importance of the candidate variables to be retained or excluded in a clinimetric index.

A third use of mathematical models is particularly interesting because the model produces the actual clinimetric index itself. Thus, in a multiple regression model such as $Y = b_0 + b_1 X_1 + b_2 X_2 + b_3 X_3 + \ldots$, the b_1, b_2, $b_3, \ldots$ coefficients represent a weight given to each of the variables X_1, X_2, $X_3, \ldots$, which can represent the components of a prognostic index. When a particular patient's data for X_1, X_2, $X_3, \ldots$ are entered into this model, the value of Y becomes a clinimetric index, predicting the patient's likelihood of survival at a particular time in the future. The clinimetric role of an index such as TNM stage is readily apparent if we predict prognosis of a patient with a particular cancer by saying that he is in **TNM Stage III,** and that patients in this stage have a **20% one-year survival rate.** The mathematical model would have a similar clinimetric role if we obtained $Y = .20$ for the estimate of one-year survival after entering the patient's data for each of the appropriate variables into the regression equation $Y = b_0 + b_1X_1 + b_2X_2 + b_3X_3 + \ldots$.

8.1.2. INFERENTIAL STATISTICS

A quite different set of mathematical models, aimed at concepts of probability rather than description, produces the P values, confidence intervals, and other inferential expressions that often appear in medical literature today. These models are used to indicate the numerical or probabilistic fragility of the descriptive statistical expressions. For example, we would surely feel more confident about the stability of a 20% value for a survival rate if it arises from numbers such as 60/300 than if the numbers are 1/5. Similarly, if Treatment A has a success rate of 50% and Treatment B has a success rate of 33%, the superiority of Treatment A seems impressive. If we learn, however, that the success rates are based on a comparison of 1/2 vs. 1/3, we would no longer be impressed. With only five people under study, the difference of 50% vs. 33% could easily arise by chance alone if the two treatments are equivalent.

The P values, confidence intervals, and other acts of inferential statistics allow estimates of the numerical role played by chance. When the P values are small enough and the confidence intervals are narrow enough, we can infer that the numerical distinctions are stable, firm, and not likely to be probabilistic caprices of random chance.

Since our main concern here is with descriptive rather than inferential statistics, the mathematical strategies used for probabilistic decisions will not be further discussed. One important point about the probabilities should be noted, however, before we return to the descriptive models. When a reduction in variance is evaluated for descriptive decisions, the evaluation usually includes the demand for "significance" in both the probabilistic as well as the descriptive attributes of the data. Nevertheless, the probabilistic demand (e.g., a satisfactory P value) is often given priority of attention. Consequently, because the P values that denote "statistical significance" are strongly affected by the size and spectrum of the group(s) under study, the decisions about *descriptive* significance may often be neglected and may sometimes be contradicted. An important descriptive difference may be dismissed because the group under study was too small to achieve "statistical significance;" and a trivial descriptive difference may be falsely magnified because it occurred in a group large enough to make the P value "significant."[55]

Thus, although a clinician wants to find descriptive biologic distinctions that hold true regardless of the size and composition of the group(s) under study, the probabilistic inferential decisions of statistical significance are data dependent and may be altered by the numbers rather than by the biologic attributes of the investigated people.

8.2. **Statistical Strategies and Models**

Statistical strategies in description almost always involve the use of a model, which is a selected mechanism for fitting the observed data with a particular point, line, or other mathematical expression. Among the expressions derived from the models are a mean (which indicates the central location of data), a correlation coefficient (which shows the association of variables), and diverse multivariate citations. A detailed description of these models can be found in textbooks of statistics. The discussion here is devoted mainly to the way in which the statistical goals of these models differ or coincide with the goals of clinimetric description.

8.2.1. REDUCTION TO A SUMMARY

The most common descriptive use of statistical techniques is to summarize a set of data. For information containing values for a single variable in each member of a group, the univariate data are reduced to such summary expressions as a mean and standard deviation. For the relationships of two variables or in multivariate data, the summaries are cited in such indexes of association as regression coefficients and correlation coefficients.

By eliminating detail, the summaries perform a splendid statistical job, but the eliminated details are often crucial for judgmental functions in clinical or biological reasoning. This elimination has been the source of many complaints—from the old laments about the "numerical method" of the nineteenth century[9] to modern-day distresses about computerized "number crunching"—that clinical decisions cannot be made on the basis of mean values for an average patient.

At this very elemental level of thought, therefore, the statistician and clinician may have strikingly different goals. The statistician wants to create summaries as acts of data reduction to remove details. The greater the amount of reduction, the greater is the apparent success of the statistical process. On the other hand, a clinician, although also interested in summarizing the data, is particularly eager to preserve details that may be important for analyzing the results and for making subsequent decisions. Unless those details are clearly identified and recognized beforehand, they may be lost when the summary statistics are created.

8.2.2. DIRECT VS. INDIRECT EXPRESSIONS

When a statistical expression such as $\overline{X} \pm s$ (the mean and standard deviation) is offered as a summary of data for a single variable, the details may be reduced, but the results are shown directly. The mean value offers a direct indication of a central location for the magnitude of the data. The standard deviation offers a direct statement about the spread of the data around the mean. As a further act of data reduction, however, we can combine these two statistical expressions into a single summary, called the *coefficient of variation* (c.v.), which is calculated as $s/\overline{X}$. The latter expression is indirect because the basic evidence is no longer visible when the two values are converted into a ratio. For example, if we are told that the c.v. is 2.5, we can assume that the data are widely spread around the mean, but we have no idea of the real values for location and spread of the data. The mean and standard deviation might be 100 ± 250, or $.01 \pm .025$.

An analogous problem constantly occurs when data are summarized with a statistical expression of association, which always presents an indirect account of the results. A coefficient of association summarizes a relationship between two (or more) variables, but does not show direct evidence of that relationship. For example, suppose the five-year survival rate was found to be 51% ($= 154/300$) for a group of people with a particular disease. Suspecting that survival depends on the clinical severity of stage of illness, the investigator wants to check the association between stage and survival. The result is reported as a correlation coefficient of $-.45$ (with $p < .001$) for the inverse relationship. Because the coefficient seems significantly high, the investigator concludes that survival is definitely affected by clinical stage of disease.

Although this conclusion is correct, the correlation coefficient offered no direct evidence, and gave only an indirect summary of the relationship. If presented, the direct evidence might be arranged in the manner displayed in the following table:

Clinical Stage	Survival Rate	
I	56/70	*(80%)*
II	55/89	*(62%)*
III	28/61	*(46%)*
IV	15/80	*(19%)*
Total	154/300	*(51%)*

The inverse relationship between stage and survival is now readily apparent. If we wanted to give a direct descriptive summary of this relationship, however, we would need an array of additional words and numbers. We might say that the results show a striking survival gradient, ranging from 80% in Stage I to 19% in Stage IV, with strong interstage gradients of 18% (from Stage I to II), 16% (from II to III), and 27% (from III to IV). Furthermore, a clinician meeting an individual patient could use these results to estimate prognosis directly. If the patient happens to be in Stage II, the chance of five-year survival is 62%. In Stage IV, the chance of five-year survival is 19%, etc. All of this additional evidence and verbiage could be eliminated with the use of a single statistical summary index, describing the correlation as −.45, but we would no longer be able to use the evidence in direct clinical interpretation and judgment.

Both the indirect and direct methods of describing the relationship between stage and survival are entirely correct and justifiable, but each method has its advantages and disadvantages. The correlation coefficient offers a major economy of expression. It summarizes the entire relationship with a single number, −.45, whereas the display of the table takes much more space, and its description requires many words and numbers. On the other hand, the correlation coefficient does not show the actual data, and its numerical value cannot be used effectively in any subsequent clinical decisions or predictions for individual patients.

Since both methods of expressing the results are useful, the two methods could be employed in a complementary manner, particularly since a computer can be programmed to produce both sets of results. Nevertheless, in many statistical approaches, the relationship is reported only with an indirect coefficient of association, and the actual evidence is not displayed. The statistical policy is useful for its economy of space and expression, but it deprives the investigator (and the reader) of direct evidence that can be examined for judgments about what actually happened.

8.2.3. PROBLEMS IN MULTIVARIATE DESCRIPTIONS

The descriptive economy of the indirect statistical coefficients seems even more attractive when multivariate information is summarized. If we wanted to examine the simultaneous relationship of survival to such multiple variables as age, hematocrit, anatomic extensiveness of the lesion, comorbidity, and several chemical measurements, as well as clinical stage of severity, the direct presentation of evidence might require an unwieldy array of tables. To form those tables, we would also have to make many arbitrary decisions about the boundaries for different categories of age, hematocrit, and the chemical measurements.

The supreme advantage of the indirect coefficients is that they seem to eliminate all these problems and judgmental decisions. With a suitable mathematical arrangement, an association coefficient will denote the relative importance of each variable, and no arbitrary decisions are needed to demarcate categories of dimensional variables. On the other hand, since no direct evidence is presented, an investigator (or reader) who wants to make judgmental decisions from the results has no specific information with which to think and work.

8.2.4. FITTING A MODEL

The mathematical models used for data reduction are usually chosen for their elegant simplicity in calculation and for their justification as mechanisms of variance reduction. For example, the mean is usually preferred over the median as a statistical central index because the mean is calculated from all the data, whereas the median is merely the middle-ranked value, and because the expression $\Sigma(X_i - K)^2$, which is used to calculate variance, has its smallest value when $K = \Sigma X_i/N$, i.e., the mean.

For similar reasons, indexes of association are calculated with a simple linear model, having the form $Y = a + bX$ or $Y = b_0 + b_1X_1 + b_2X_2 + b_3X_3 + b_4X_4 + \ldots$. The simple linear model is preferred because it is standardized. If we wanted to use a quadratic expression such as $Y = a + bX + cX^2$ or some other model such as $Y = b_0 + b_1X_1 + b_2\sqrt{X_2} + b_3X_3^4 + b_4e^{-X_4} + \ldots$, the decisions about which terms to include and how to include them would no longer be simple or standardized. With the linear model of arrangement, the coefficients that become the indexes of association are calculated with another standardized technique, the method of least squares, which usually also leads to a maximum reduction in the numerical variance of the system.

The mathematical principles cannot be faulted, but the biologic consequences are not always proper or correct. Despite the statistical advantages of the mean in reducing variance, the median is often more suitable as a *clinical* index of central tendency than a mean. In other circumstances, a linear model may fail to show a consistent, close relationship that is best demonstrated with a non-linear model. In the analysis of certain multiple-variable relationships, a logistic model is often preferred to a linear model (as noted in Section 8.3.3) because the latter may produce impossible values when subsequently applied to individual patients.

In all these activities, the fitted mathematical models retain their theoretical elegance and pragmatic accomplishments in variance reduction. The decision that the model does not fit and that some other model is needed almost always requires clinical rather than mathematical reasoning.

8.2.5. THE PRINCIPLE OF VARIANCE REDUCTION

The idea of using variance reduction as a criterion of statistical accomplishment is entirely sound. Like other statistical mechanisms, it is standardized and it offers the best general approach to decisions about the fit of a model. In many biologic circumstances, however, the investigator's goal may differ from the standardized general approach.

For example, suppose we want to develop a staging system for making prognostic predictions in a group of patients having the overall survival rate of $150/300 = 50\%$. We can use two staging systems, depending on either Variable A or Variable B, each of which has three categories. With Variable A, the survival results are as follows:

$$a_1: 80/100 = 80\%$$
$$a_2: 50/100 = 50\%$$
$$a_3: 20/100 = 20\%$$

With Variable B, the results are:

$$b_1: 20/20 = 100\%$$
$$b_2: 130/260 = 50\%$$
$$b_3: 0/20 = 0\%$$

If forced to choose between these two systems of staging, the statistical model would prefer System A because it produces a greater reduction in the variance of the data.* On the other hand, a clinician might strongly prefer System B because it allows a relatively certain prediction of survival for the 20 patients in Category b_1, and of non-survival for the 20 patients in Category b_3. For the 260 patients in Category b_2, the clinician might then seek some other mechanism (such as Variable A) to help improve predictive accuracy.

A second problem in the variance-reduction criterion is that it depends completely on the distribution and sample size of the particular data that have been entered into the mathematical model. If certain groups or phenomena are under-represented in the data, their importance may be missed or overlooked because they are not large enough numerically to produce variance reductions that are statistically significant. For example, suppose the group just cited had the same proportionate composition, but suppose it

*Using the formula $\Sigma n_i p_i q_i$ for the overall variance in each system, the result in System A is: $(100)(80/100)(20/100)+(100)(50/100)(50/100)+(100)(20/100)(80/100) = 57$. The corresponding result for System B is: $(20)(20/20)(0/20)+(260)(130/260)(130/260)+(20)(0/20)(20/20) = 65$.

contained 30 rather than 300 patients. The survival results for Variable A would be a_1: $8/10 = 80\%$; a_2: $5/10 = 50\%$; and a_3: $2/10 = 20\%$. The results for Variable B would be b_1: $2/2 = 100\%$; b_2: $13/26 = 50\%$; b_3: $0/2 = 0\%$. The proportionate reduction in the original variance would be the same in both systems, and the prognostic importance of categories of b_1 and b_3 would still be shown in the second system; but the second system might now be rejected from consideration. Because of the small numbers, its results would not be statistically significant, whereas the first system (for Variable A), having a better distribution of its small numbers, would successfully achieve significance.

Because the variance-reduction process is strongly data dependent, the same biologic phenomena may receive different statistical descriptions according to the distribution and size of data in the particular group under study. The problems of this type of data-dependent analysis are often manifested by the inconsistencies found when the results of a multivariate mathematical model are applied to a different group of patients at a later date or in a different medical setting. The inconsistencies can be distressing because the biologic goal in clinical description is to find variables whose descriptive power persists regardless of the composition of the particular group of people to whom the descriptions are applied. This goal may not be achieved if the selected variables are altered by the numerical rather than the clinical or biologic attributes of a particular group whose data are used for the mathematical analysis.

None of the cited problems detracts from the magnificent accomplishments of statistical models. The problems merely indicate that the mathematical goals are aimed at eliminating details, using standardized models, and producing maximum reductions of variance in the available data. If these goals happen to coincide with the clinician's goals, the mathematical models will be splendid. On the other hand, if the clinician wants to preserve details, observe direct evidence of relationships, choose descriptions that will be specifically fitted to specific relationships, and arrive at conclusions that are clinically both cogent and consistent, the conventional mathematical goals will not always be satisfactory.

8.3. Diversity of Choices and Policies in Multivariate Models

When multiple variables are candidates for combination in a clinical index, a decision-making mechanism must be established to choose, weight, and combine the cogent variables. If the mechanism used for this process is clinical judgment, the process may sometimes work very well, but the judgment often may be applied in an inconsistent, unstandardized, or even capricious manner. The great appeal of multivariate mathematical models is that they offer a standardized mechanism for this process. No matter who uses the model, it should give the same results for the same set of data.

Despite the appeal of a standardized mechanism, however, the use of the mathematical models merely transfers the judgmental decisions from one intellectual location to another. Someone who wants to use the models must first decide which model to choose among the many that are available and must then make a series of other judgments about policy options for the actual operation of each model. Once chosen and programmed, a model will do its work in a consistent standardized manner, and the role of judgment in choosing among models and policy options may be overlooked.

The rest of this section contains an outline of the available multivariate models and an account of the options that must be chosen in policy decisions for the type of output scale, the direction of the association, the rating of the dependent variable, and the mechanism used to denote the importance of component variables.

8.3.1. SCORE AND CLUSTER SCALES FOR OUTPUT

Like a clinimetric index, a mathematical model of association can generate its output as a score or cluster. The most frequently used and well-known statistical models produce an arithmetical score. For example, in the model for a simple correlation or regression of two variables, the relationship of one variable, Y, to another variable, X, is expressed as the score obtained in the linear model $Y = a + bX$. For multivariate associations, this linear model is expanded to the form of a "surface," $Y = b_0 + b_1X_1 + b_2X_2 + b_3X_3 + \ldots$. Among such arithmetical-score models are multiple linear regression, factor analysis, and several others to be cited later.

Because these additive linear models have been so attractive, relatively little statistical attention has been given to the type of clustered categories that are commonly used in clinical thought. In recent years, however, with computers to help in the difficult number crunching, several models for categorical clusters have been developed. The procedures have been called *cluster analysis*[81] by statisticians, *numerical taxonomy*[144] by quantitative biologists, and *automated interaction detection*[145] by social scientists. Unlike the arithmetical-score models, the cluster procedures operate in a relatively pragmatic manner, unaccompanied by a strong, well-established set of theoretical principles about linear, log-linear, polynomial, or other conceptual models for the data. Consequently, the cluster procedures are not mathematically popular and are seldom advocated for clinical usage.

A clinician who wants to form a clustered-category multivariate index can sometimes use an arithmetic-score model—as noted later in Section 8.3.4—to screen the data and identify important variables. Aided by the results of the mathematical screening, the clinician may then make judgmental decisions about optimal categories and clusters. In most circumstances, however, a mathematical procedure is programmed to do its work from start to finish, accepting input data and producing an output equation, score, or cluster, with no human intervention during the intermediate stages.

Because the contents of multivariate clusters may be difficult to remember, clinicians sometimes assign numerical ratings to the categories and convert them into the type of scored cluster that was illustrated in Section 3.4.2.2.

8.3.2. DEPENDENT AND INTERDEPENDENT DIRECTIONS

An important judgment in choosing a model is to decide whether the direction of the association is dependent or interdependent. The direction is dependent if we believe that one of the variables is distinctly affected by the other(s). For example, if we were examining the relationship between blood pressure and weight, we would assume that blood pressure depends on weight, but not that weight depends on blood pressure. On the other hand, for the relationship between hematocrit and hemoglobin levels, we would regard the two variables as interdependent, with no belief that one depends on the other.

The choice of direction is particularly important for choosing the format of a regression model. Thus, if Y = blood pressure and X = weight, we would express the dependency relationship in the form of $Y = a + bX$; and b would be the *regression coefficient* for the regression Y on X. Alternatively, however, if we regarded weight as dependent on blood pressure, we would have formed the equation as $X = a' + b'Y$. In the latter instance b' would be the regression coefficient for the regression of X (weight) on Y (blood pressure).

In situations where we want to know about the interdependency of two variables, such as hemoglobin and hematocrit, without specifying a direction for the relationship, we would use the *correlation coefficient*, r, as the statistical index of association. Because r is calculated from the two possible regression coefficients as $\sqrt{bb'}$, it yields an intermediate result that is their geometric mean. Another virtue of r is that its values lie between -1 and $+1$, and are unaffected by the units of original measurement. Thus, if we expressed weight in kg. instead of lb., the original regression coefficient between blood pressure and weight would be altered, but the correlation coefficient would be unchanged. For this reason, r is sometimes called the *standardized regression coefficient*.

8.3.2.1. *The Role of r^2*

The most important function of r, however, is the role of r^2 in helping indicate the success of the mathematical model. If we used $\overline{Y}$ to fit each of the Y_i values with their mean, the residual group variance in the system would be the sum of the squared deviations around the mean, expressed as $S_{yy} = \Sigma(Y_i - \overline{Y})^2$. When we fit each of the observed Y_i values with a different value, $\hat{Y}_i$, which is estimated from the associated X_i values as the straight line $\hat{Y}_i = a + bX_i$, the residual group variance in the system will be the sum of the squared deviations around the line. These would be expressed as $S_r = \Sigma(Y_i - \hat{Y}_i)^2$. By comparing the original value for S_{yy} with the subsequent value for S_r, we appraise the success of the straight line in fitting the data and "explaining" the original variance. If Y indeed has a good linear relationship to X, we would expect the original variance in the system to be substantially reduced. This proportionate reduction in variance is calculated and expressed as:

$$r^2 = \frac{S_{yy} - S_r}{S_{yy}}$$

Thus, if the line fits particularly well, the value of S_r will be small and r^2 will be close to 1. If the line does not fit well, S_r will be almost as large as S_{yy} and r^2 will be close to 0.

This same principle is used in all other additive-score models of statistical association. The accomplishment of the model, or of individual variables in the model, is determined by noting the proportion of the original variance that has been reduced or explained.

8.3.2.2. *Availability of a Dependent Variable*

Although r^2 (or its corresponding multivariate analog, R^2) can be calculated regardless of the direction of the relationship, a specific direction is chosen when a particular variable is used as a criterion or target in the research. For example, if we have data on patients' definitive diagnoses, and if we want to develop a mathematical model to see how the diagnoses are related to symptoms and various laboratory tests, the definitive diagnoses would be the dependent variable, "predicted" by the symptoms and laboratory data. A similar arrangement would be used if the patient's three-year survival status, as alive or dead, is used as a target or dependent variable to be predicted from current symptoms and laboratory data.

In other types of research, however, a particular dependent variable is not chosen (or available) as a target. Instead, the multiple variables are examined for their interrelationship or interdependency with one another. Given a set of variables that denote different features of psychic or social behavior in a group of people, we might want to see which of those features are highly correlated with one another rather than with a specific outcome variable. The mathematical models of *factor analysis, principal component analysis,* and *cluster analysis* are often used for this type of activity, which is particularly common in psychosocial research. One of the goals is to see whether the existing variables can be reduced to a smaller number of factors, principal components, or clusters that are characterized by a close association of the component parts. For example, if data for a group of people are expressed in the six variables X_1, X_2, X_3, X_4, X_5, and X_6, we might find that the variance in the system is best explained by two factors, cited as:

$$v_1 = 0.4X_1 + 0.7X_4 - 0.3X_5$$

and

$$v_2 = 1.7X_2 - 0.4X_3$$

These two factors, expressed as combinations of the existing variables, would allow us to reduce the original six variables $(X_1, \ldots, X_6)$ to the two final "variables," v_1 and v_2, while simultaneously reducing the variance of the system. Because this variance reduction may be regarded as an important explanatory power of the factors, they may be retained in future research, thus becoming descriptive indexes that were generated by a multivariate mathematical model.

When categorical clusters are desired rather than additive combinations of variables, the corresponding approach uses *cluster analysis* or, more recently, the *log-linear analysis of multidimensional contingency tables.*[10]

8.3.3. RATING OF THE DEPENDENT VARIABLE

In contrast to the factor-analysis situation, many clinical analyses have an available dependent variable, often provided by data about diagnoses or prognostic outcomes. The data analyst must then choose among several multivariate models for expressing the dependency relationship. The choice will often be determined by the particular type of rating or other scale in which the dependent variable has been expressed.

The best-known model, *multiple linear regression,* has been particularly popular in epidemiologic or clinical research where the dependent variable is commonly an event cited as **absent** or **present.** The event may be life (or death) or the development of a particular disease at a future point in time. Because the event is coded as **0** or **1,** the clinimetric index that emerges from the regression equation is a probability value, predicting the likelihood of that event. Thus, an expression such as y (= survival) = b_0+b_1(age)+b_2(gender)+b_3 (clinical severity)+ . . . in a multiple linear regression equation may yield .23 as the probability of survival for a particular patient. Since probabilities must lie between 0 and 1, the equation will produce bizarre results when it sometimes yields a value below 0 or above 1 for the data of an individual patient.

To avoid this problem, a logistic transformation can be used to constrain the dependent variable so that its result always lies between 0 and 1 in a mathematical process called multiple logistic regression. Its results for coefficients and variables often resemble those of multiple linear regression, although the weighting coefficients for each variable are calculated with a different principle (since the least-squares linear strategy is not applicable). The coefficients must be interpreted as odds ratios rather than as linear weights.

Multiple logistic regression can be applied only when the dependent variable is expressed in binary form, but multiple linear regression has been applied to manage dependent variables that are binary, ordinal, or dimensional. Neither of these two models, however, can deal with a dependent variable that has an unranked nominal scale, such as *type of diagnosis*. For the latter purpose, the customary mathematical model is *discriminant function analysis*. Discriminant function analysis can also be applied to binary dependent variables, where it yields results identical to those obtained with multiple linear regression.

Two other multivariate models are also available for application to dependent variables. The proportional hazards model, often called Cox regression, can be applied when the dependent variable is a complete curve of duration of survival over time, rather than a binary survival for an event at a single point in time. The AID (automated interaction detector) model developed by social scientists can be applied if the goal is to develop targeted clusters, rather than scores, for predicting an outcome event.[145]

8.3.4. IMPORTANCE OF COMPONENT VARIABLES

When component variables are entered into the multivariate models that form clinimetric indexes, decisions are regularly made about eliminating unimportant variables and denoting the importance of those that remain. In a targeted cluster index, the importance of the retained components can be shown by the associated value of the target event. For example, if **TNM Stages I, II,** and **III** were produced by a multivariate model, the quantitative importance of the stages would be shown by the associated median survival times in a gradient such as 12.4 mos., 8.3 mos., and 2.0 mos. If the index is constructed by a score such as $Y = b_0+b_1X_1+b_2X_2+b_3X_3+\ldots$ the values of the b_i coefficients can be expressed as "standard regression coefficients" or as "standardized weights," which will show each variable's relative importance in the assigned task of explaining variance.

Before each component of the index was retained, however, some of the candidate variables may have been eliminated. In both the cluster and the score procedures, the eliminations depend on the way a particular variable (or its component categories) reduces variance in the system. A technique called *stepwise regression* has become particularly popular for eliminating candidate variables in indexes constructed as a score. In the "step-up" process, all independent candidates are first examined in a simple regression to find the single variable that provides the best reduction in variance. The next regression equation begins with this "best" variable entered as the first variable; and all other candidates are individually tested for their variance reduction as the second independent variable. The best of these candidates is then entered into the equation as a second independent variable; and the process is reiterated in the third step with each remaining candidate tested for best reduction in variance as a third independent variable. The process continues, incrementally building up the number of variables in the equation, until no additional variable produces an adequate (i.e., statistically significant) reduction in variance. The process then ends, having eliminated the unimportant variables and having assigned suitable weighting coefficients to the important ones that were retained. The process can also be operated in a reverse "step-down" manner.

With or without a logistic transformation or a stepwise operation, multiple regression has become frequently used to examine multivariate data in search of prognostic or risk factors for outcome events in clinical and epidemiologic research. The results often serve directly as a clinimetric index that can be applied either to make predictions for individual patients, or to help analyze complex statistical studies of therapeutic agents. For example, the index attained with a multiple regression analysis of variables in a series of patients with chest pain[133] was later used (and evaluated) as a guide for the clinical decisions made in a new group of patients.[134] Analogous multivariate indexes have been applied to adjust for "confounding factors" that may lead to pre-therapeutic imbalances of the groups of patients studied in a randomized (or nonrandomized) trial.

Because the multivariate regression model produces a score that has no overt biologic content, efforts are sometimes made to convert the results into a simpler arrangement that is biologically easier to understand. For this purpose, the individual variables of the regression equation are demarcated into ordinal or binary categories, each of which is assigned an arbitrary numerical rating based on the size of the associated weighting coefficient. The numerical ratings for each category in a particular patient will then resemble the components of an Apgar score. They will be individually easy to recognize and understand, and the sum of the added ratings will form a type of scored cluster.

For example, Feigenbaum et al.[36] used stepwise discriminant function analysis to identify six variables that had cogently predicted the outcome of patients with rheumatoid arthritis. Instead of preserving the six variables and their coefficients as an equation expressed in the form of $b_0+b_1x_1+b_2x_2+\ldots+b_6x_6$, the investigators converted the variables to a simple categorical scoring system. A score of 2 points was given for rheumatoid factor positivity and for swelling of two or more joints in the upper extremity. A score of 1 point was given for each of four other features (Raynaud's-like symptoms, malaise or weakness, white race, and female gender). The sum of these six numerical ratings formed a "simple arithmetic prediction score," ranging from **0** to **8,** that correlated well with the patients' outcomes.

Because the biologic categories are clearly identified, with simple ratings and a simple addition process to form the output score, the scored cluster arrangement is much simpler and easier to comprehend than an unadorned regression formula.

8.4. The Underlying Mathematical Judgments

With the easy availability of package programs that can readily execute the complex multivariate calculations on a digital computer, mathematical models have become frequently applied in both psychosocial and medical research. Their great appeal is that they can avoid the problems, difficulties, and inconsistencies that arise when judgment is used to choose variables, assign ratings, and form aggregations. The mathematical process is specified and standardized so that it always does the same thing in the same way.

To conduct a specified standardized process is obviously appealing to scientists, but the overt judgments eliminated during the mathematical process are transferred to a series of more subtle conceptual judgments made before the process begins. Although well known to statistical consultants, these conceptual judgments may not be recognized or clearly understood by the clinical collaborators.

8.4.1. CHOICE OF A MODEL

The first conceptual judgment is the choice of a particular mathematical model. Many different models are available—each with its own well-constructed logic and pattern of operation. Although several models might be applicable to the same set of data, and although each choice might be individually justified, the different models do not necessarily yield the same results for choices of variables and for the weights assigned to coefficients.[155] In a phenomenon analogous to observer variability, the results may sometimes show striking disparities when the same set of data is processed by two different mathematical models. Because the statistical results are so data dependent, substantial differences may be found—although the basic biologic issues remain unchanged—when the same model is applied to a different group of people.

8.4.2. VIOLATION OF UNDERLYING ASSUMPTIONS

A second judgment involves the violation of certain mathematical requirements for the basic logic of the model. In the assumptions made for the mathematical analyses, the data are often required to have a multivariate Gaussian distribution—i.e., the data must be Gaussian in each variable as well as in the simultaneous arrangement of variables. This requirement is seldom, if ever, fulfilled by the data of the groups studied in clinical and epidemiologic research. The mathematical models are generally regarded as "robust," i.e., able to work well even when the basic requirements are violated. Judgment is needed, however, to decide when and whether the robustness may fail, so that the model becomes inappropriate.

8.4.3. SELECTION OF INTERACTION TERMS

A third judgment requires decisions about when and how to put interaction terms into the mathematical model. Statisticians use the word *interaction* for what clinicians might call a synergistic or antagonistic effect when two or more categories are conjoined in a cluster. Thus, a group of **tall old men** or **short young women** might have results that are strikingly higher (or lower) than might be expected from the trend of the data found for individual categories of age, height, and gender. This type of conjoined effect is well known in clinical experience. For example, the survival rate for patients with acute myocardial infarction might be 50% if the patient is in shock or 50% if the patient has acute pulmonary edema. If these two attributes are independent, a mathematical model might expect the survival rate to be 25% when both attributes are present. In clinical reality, however, the survival rate is usually 0% when the patient has both shock and pulmonary edema.

Because interaction terms are not included in the standard format of the mathematical models, anyone who is interested in the possibility of interactions must anticipate what they might be and then enter them into the model. Thus, if X_1 = gender and X_2 = age, the interaction of gender and age would be entered as an X_1X_2 term in the equation $Y = b_0+b_1X_1+b_2X_2+b_3X_1X_2+\ldots$. If we anticipate an interaction of three variables—gender, age, and height—and if X_3 = height, the added interaction term would be $X_1X_2X_3$. Although the mathematical models can handle all of the interaction terms that might be entered, the computation process would be extensive and the results would be extraordinarily difficult to interpret if—as a matter of routine operation—interaction terms were entered for all the pairs, triplets, quartets, and higher order interactions that could be explored in a multivariate analysis.

Consequently, judgmental decisions are needed about when to look for interactions, and which ones and how many to look for. Although interactions are constantly checked when clustered categories are formed by clinical judgment, none of the conventional mathematical models is programmed to do this job routinely. The only routine mathematical approach in current usage is the unconventional technique used in the non-linear, computerized algorithm of the AID[145] (automated interaction detector) procedure.

8.4.4. CHOICE OF OPERATING PARAMETERS

The fourth set of judgments involves the choice of "operating parameters" for the computer programs that carry out the selected mathematical models. At various steps in the program, decisions must be made about statistically significant reductions in variance. The level chosen for statistical significance (commonly set at $P = .05$) will determine which variables become entered, deleted, or retained in the process. Since these P values depend on the size and pattern of the data, important biologic phenomena, as discussed in Section 8.2.5, may be dismissed because they do not achieve the selected level of significance.

8.4.5. CHOICE OF ELEMENTAL VARIABLES AND UNIONS

A fifth level of judgment involves the choice of elemental or transformed variables that are entered in the analysis. No mathematical model can make the decisions that transform isolated elemental variables into sensible biologic "unions." For example, a mathematical model will accept and process data for three individual binary variables—metastasis to bone, metastasis to brain, and metastasis to liver—without recognizing that the three variables can be effectively transformed into a clustered union, distant metastasis. If the union is not previously formed by judgment and specifically entered into the analysis, and if data are too sparse for each of the three single variables, the effects of distant metastasis may be unrecognized in the analysis and in the results.

8.4.6. CHOICE OF CODING FOR DATA

A sixth level of judgment occurs when dimensional or ordinal variables are partitioned into coding arrangements that prepare the data for analysis. If a dimensional variable such as age is coded in ordinal categories, such as **0–20, 21–30, 31–40,** etc., the analytic results can be affected by the number of categories and boundaries of each category in the partition. An analogous effect can occur if we partition an ordinal variable, such as *severity of illness,* into 3, 5, 7, or more graded categories.

8.4.7. INTERPRETATION OF RESULTS

Finally, the last set of judgments involves the interpretation of results. Because complex biologic phenomena are almost never observed or contemplated in the form of an added-score mathematical model, a clinician may have major problems in trying to understand and interpret the mathematical expressions. The ingenuity of data analysts always allows an interpretation to be made, but the biologic meaning may be highly dubious, particularly if the observed variables and coefficients are biologically unstable, having emerged from quirks in the model and data rather than from true biologic distinctions.

The main point of these comments is that despite the splendid accomplishments of mathematical models, the clinical and statistical collaborators often have different policies for different goals. Both sets of policies and goals involve judgments, but the clinical judgments are readily apparent during the selection and processing of data, whereas the mathematical judgments are sometimes obscured by the complicated statistical procedures and technical expressions. To achieve more successful collaboration in the development of clinimetric indexes, both sets of collaborators can overtly state their policies, recognize the conflicting competition that may sometimes arise among the policies, and develop satisfactory methods of establishing priorities to resolve the conflicts.

Chapter 9

The Goals of Psychosocial Methods

The choice of component variables for an index, as discussed in Chapter 4, is affected by distinctive differences in the way that clinicians and psychosocial scientists make observations and collect information in their routine activities. Clinicians regularly obtain highly personal data, direct evidence of observed phenomena, and many additional kinds of information that corroborate the clinical observations. Psychosocial scientists, on the other hand, will sometimes deliberately avoid a direct personal interrogation, will often seek extrinsic evidence for phenomena, and cannot routinely depend on additional outside sources of "validation." Seeking a simple, sensible description for a phenomenon that is an accepted construct, clinicians will often choose the cogent variables at the beginning of the research by dissecting the intuition with which the phenomenon has been previously observed and appraised. Psychosocial scientists will often choose the cogent variables by working in the reverse direction. An array of multiple items is first assembled as candidates, and the cogent variables (and sometimes the selected constructs) emerge from this array after the results have been analyzed.

These distinctions in ordinary styles of professional activity are also reflected in the two main strategic goals of psychosocial theory for constructing and evaluating indexes. Not having the dimensional data that clinicians regularly obtain from laboratory tests, psychosocial investigators want to construct indexes that resemble the dimensional scales used in other forms of scientific measurement. Without other sources of data to provide informal corroborations of the observed evidence, psychosocial investigators want to validate the indexes formally, with rigorous statistical tests of "reliability" and "validity." The theory is thus aimed at dimensionality as a goal in measurement, and standardization as a goal in science.

Clinicians are not familiar with the idea of using a theory to formulate indexes. Many clinicians who develop indexes may rely on individual judgment, consensus panels, or expert consultants, but are unaware of any formal theoretical principles for clinimetric activities. Despite the absence of formal principles, however, clinicians often have a counterpart—although different—set of -metric goals. In construction, clinicians may deliberately create scales that lack dimensional characteristics; and in evaluation, clinicians may often focus more on qualitative issues in sensibility than on statistical calculations of reliability and validity.

These different emphases by clinicians and psychosocial scientists may not create any conflicts if the two groups study different phenomena. When a clinician develops an index for angina pectoris and a psychosocial scientist develops an index for ethnic prejudice, each investigator's preferred approach can be applied separately without any competition and sometimes without any awareness that alternative approaches exist. During the past two decades, however, clinicians and psychosocial scientists have increasingly studied the same phenomena, and have often collaborated in the research. Many of the rating scales now used by psychiatric (and non-psychiatric) physicians to describe anxiety, hostility, and other emotions or behaviors were originally developed by clinical psychologists. Other indexes developed in recent years for disability, functional capacity, quality of life, and satisfaction with care— topics that concern both medical clinicians and psychosocial scientists—have been the product of direct collaboration among workers in the two domains. This type of collaboration will doubtlessly increase as renewed attention is given to the description of important clinical, personal, familial, and other humanistic phenomena that have not been previously cited as analyzable data in medical care.

Clinicians and psychosocial scientists will therefore need to be better acquainted with one another's different basic approaches in the construction of indexes. The purpose of this chapter is to outline the theory that clinicians may encounter as the goals and strategies of psychosocial consultants. Chapter 10, which follows, will then provide an analogous outline of clinimetric principles that have not been hitherto expressed as "theory."

9.1. Goals of the Output Scale

In preparing the elemental scales that express data for component variables, clinicians often begin with the natural ways in which the phenomenon has been observed and described. The challenge is to convert the unspecified or intuitive process of expression into a more formal arrangement. The basic activities may require the development of new rating scales for component variables, and transformations of basic data from one scale of expression to another. After the components are appropriately expressed, they are then combined into an output scale.

In choosing the output scales, clinicians will often be satisfied with non-dimensional citations. An index that provides diagnostic criteria may be expressed in such binary categories as **present/absent** or in the nominal titles of different diseases. An index of relative magnitude may be cited in ordinal grades, such as **1+, 2+, 3+, 4+**. A composite index, such as the Apgar score, may produce results that are not unique, with the same individual score (such as **5**) often emerging from various mixtures of ratings for the individual components.

Clinicians are willing to accept these relatively soft arrangements of output scales because they satisfy the desired purpose and because so many other forms of hard dimensional data are readily available in clinical practice. In psychosocial research, however, the investigator usually has little or no pertinent information that is expressed in hard dimensions and may therefore want to create indexes and output scales that come as close as possible to the hard scientific ideal of dimensional measurement. This ideal obviously cannot be perfectly achieved with scales created from arbitrary ratings, but vigorous efforts can be made to approximate it. For the approximation, psychosocial scientists may aim at three distinctive goals—unidimensionality, monotonic patterns, and equal intervals between categories—which are discussed in the next three subsections.

9.1.1. UNIDIMENSIONALITY

Any output scale that produces a single score or categorical rating contributes an additional "dimension" to the total data, but the dimensionality of the output scale itself refers to the number of different variables (or dimensions) that are aggregated to form the scale. The Apgar score, for example, contains a multi-dimensional aggregate of five different variables. A scale for measuring temperature would be unidimensional, but a composite index such as the wind-chill factor has two component dimensions.

When the output is expressed in a global scale, the result may seem uni-dimensional because the constituent variables have not been overtly identified and stipulated. When an apparently uni-dimensional global rating, such as **excellent, good, fair,** or **poor** for condition of newborn baby, is dissected and converted into the specified components of an Apgar Score, however, the multi-dimensional input becomes apparent.

In many psychosocial indexes, the goal is to create a uni-dimensional scale that describes a single well-delineated attribute without any admixture of other attributes. The idea is to isolate something, such as ethnic prejudice or intelligence, without including contributions from other entities, such as political beliefs or educational status. If the index is formed as a combination of multiple items, the unidimensionality of the items can be checked (as noted later in Chapter 11) with statistical calculations of "internal consistency." The idea is to demonstrate that the items are relatively homogeneous (and therefore unidimensional) because they all "measure the same thing."

This quest for a unidimensional scale is a quite reasonable goal in scientific measurement, but it may not always be what a clinician wants. In particular, when constructing a composite index such as the Apgar Score or the TNM stages of cancer, the clinician deliberately includes the many different variables that make the result multi-dimensional. In such circumstances, the unidimensional and multi-dimensional goals will be in direct conflict. The scientific goal of reducing a complex phenomenon to single dimensions will be incompatible with the descriptive goal of summarizing multivariate complexity.

9.1.2 MONOTONIC PATTERN

The word *monotonic* refers to an ordered array in which each successive category is progressively larger (or smaller) than its predecessor. The sequence of **mild, moderate, extreme** is monotonic, but **moderate, mild, extreme** is not. When two ranked variables have a direct relationship, we often expect both sets of values to be monotonic. Suppose the rates of success in relation to baseline clinical severity are mild, **80%**; moderate, **55%**; and extreme, **20%**. In this situation, the outcome data and the baseline categories are both monotonic, but they would not be if the success rates were mild, **60%**; moderate, **35%**; and extreme, **85%**.

In most multivariable indexes, the components have monotonic rating scales, expressed in binary, ordinal, quasi-dimensional, or dimensional values. When these individual monotonic variables are combined into a single output scale, however, the categories of the output scale may not maintain a consistent monotonicity in the component elements. For example, a baby with an Apgar score of **5** may outrank a baby with a score of **6** in several constituent categories. Thus, a baby with an **Apgar 5** produced by 1+1+1+1+1 has a lower rank in three categories and a higher rank in two categories than a baby whose **Apgar 6** occurs as 2+2+2+0+0.

A consistent pattern of monotonicity is easy to achieve if the scale is unidimensional, containing only one variable, such as age, blood pressure, weight, or briskness of reflexes. If several variables are combined into a single output scale, however, the output scale may itself seem monotonic, but the constituent elements may not have a consistently monotonic pattern. We cannot be sure that a person in a higher category of the output scale will have higher ratings for each constituent element than a person in a lower category.

If certain variables are assigned a pre-emptive importance, the index can be given a *hierarchical* structure, but the hierarchy may not produce a consistently monotonic pattern for all the elements of the index. For example, the stages of the TNM staging system are hierarchically organized according to anatomic evidence of the cancer's dissemination. A patient who is in category **M2** will be assigned to **Stage III,** regardless of the individual values of T and N, and may have more favorable ratings for T and N than someone who is in the "better" **Stage I** or **II.**

Psychosocial scientists try to get monotonic patterns by making suitable choices of attributes to be emphasized. For example, in creating a rating scale for magnitude of ethnic prejudice, we might assume that someone who does not want a member of a particular ethnic group as a neighbor would almost surely not want such a person as a close friend. Someone who rejected the possibility of friendship would almost surely reject the idea of marriage to a member of that group. Consequently, we could construct a distinctively monotonic scale by using the successive categories of **would not want to marry, would not want as friend, would not want as neighbor.** The scale has included different concepts—such as marriage, friendship, and neighbor-liness—but monotonicity is preserved because the concepts act as ranked categories, not as individual component variables.

For many clinimetric indexes that provide composite summaries, a consistently monotonic pattern may be unnecessary. The goal may be simply to combine several different variables into a single composite expression that will suitably encompass all of them. If an Apgar Score of **6** offers a useful summary of a baby's clinical condition, we may not be concerned about the individual values or relative ranks of each of the five constituent scores. If we want to know those individual values, we can look for them as individual ratings on the component scales.

The clinical goal of a composite summary may thus come in conflict with the psychosocial goal of a uniquely monotonic pattern. Trying to get a unidimensional index, the psychosocial scientist wants the monotonic pattern to help indicate that the scale measures gradations of a single attribute rather than unspecified mixtures of several attributes. Although the quest for a monotonic pattern can be readily justified in psychosocial policy, the goal may not be needed (and may lead to unsatisfactory results) if the clinimetric aim is merely to combine multiple constituents.

9.1.3. EQUI-INTERVAL CATEGORIES

Accustomed to communicating in such phrases as **4+ sick, moderate dyspnea,** and **slightly enlarged,** clinicians are quite prepared to accept rating scales that produce an ordinal set of graded categories. The scales may come supplied with graded numbers, such as TNM stages, or with arbitrarily assigned numerical ratings, such as Apgar Scores; and the numerical values may sometimes be used as quasi-dimensional data from which means and standard deviations are calculated; but no one regards the scales as having truly dimensional data.

In many psychosocial indexes, however, the goal is to resemble the dimensional characteristics of measurably equal intervals between adjacent categories. Since this goal must be attained from basic data that are not dimensional, the investigator may need to use heroic methods, which are often unnecessary in ordinal scales, to establish and demonstrate the equi-interval accomplishment.

The equi-interval approach, which is used in the Thurstone scales discussed later in Section 9.2.2, may sometimes be quite justified for certain psychosocial indexes, but the policy may be difficult to apply, and it can lead to unnecessary extra efforts as well as unsatisfactory results when applied inappropriately in constructing clinimetric indexes. An example of some of the problems created by this policy is presented later in Section 9.4.

9.2. Theory of Construction

In pursuing the foregoing goals, psychosocial scientists can use several policies as theory for the construction of indexes. The indexes are often labeled eponymically according to Thurstone, Likert, or Guttman, who originated the three main theories that are outlined in the sections that follow.

9.2.1. GENERAL OPERATIONAL POLICIES

All three psychosocial policies have several basic similarities. They all use the analytic-selection method of choosing variables. The investigator begins with a large group (often 100 or more) of items containing elemental statements with which respondents are asked to denote degrees of agreement, disagreement, or other reactions. The elemental statements are submitted to a panel of judges assembled by the investigator, who then uses a separate combination of judgmental and mathematical models to analyze the responses.

The three types of psychosocial theories differ in their ordinal, monotonic, or equi-interval goals; in the types of constituent scales used for soliciting responses to the elemental item statements; and in the methods used for analyzing responses to the items.

9.2.2. THURSTONE SCALES

As one of the pioneers in developing psychosocial scales, Thurstone[151] was particularly eager to get an equi-interval set of output categories. For this purpose, a long list of elemental statements is chosen to cover a wide range of possible attitudes about the phenomenon under consideration. Each elemental statement (or "item") is then rated by each member of a panel of judges. The judges, choosing a rating from an eleven-category set of ordinal grades, are supposed to indicate not their own attitude to each statement, but the inference that might be drawn about the attitude of someone who agrees or disagrees with the statement.

For example, suppose we want to construct a scale concerned with admiration for doctors. Someone who agrees with a statement that says "I don't do anything a doctor says unless I get a second opinion" might be rated by a judge as having a quite low degree of admiration. On the other hand, agreement with a statement such as "Doctors have been licensed to practice medicine" might be rated as neutral, since the statement contains no particular aspects of admiration or disdain.

The ratings given by the group of selected judges are then summarized to note the median value and dispersion of the ratings for each statement. Statements that received a wide range of dispersion in the judges' ratings are eliminated, thus preserving only the elements that have a "compact" median value. From the remaining "compactly-rated" statements, the investigator chooses a set of statements whose median values will span the range of 1.5, 2.0, 2.5, ..., 10.0, 10.5. The median values become the scores assigned to each statement.

When the scale is applied in subsequent usage, the respondent is asked to agree or disagree (in binary fashion) with each of the submitted statements. The output score is determined as the median of the previously established scores for the statements with which the respondent agrees. For example, in a procedure containing five statements, the respondent might agree with statements whose assigned scores are 8.5, 8.0, 7.5, 7.5, and 3.5. The respondent would then be given the median rating of 7.5. If everything has worked well, the respondent will agree only with statements that have similar scores, thus giving the respondent a compact median value. The resulting final score should locate the respondent in a reasonably precise position on the equi-interval scale. If the respondent agrees with statements that have a wide range of scores, either the respondent or the scale is inconsistent.

Because the Thurstone scale presumably produces a single point on a continuum, it is often called a *differential* scale. Because of the difficulties of creating differential equi-interval scales that will work effectively, Thurstone scales have not had widespread popularity.

9.2.3. LIKERT SCALES

Likert's goals[112] were to create a distinctively ordinal scale rather than an equi-interval scale, and to eliminate a scoring system based on inferences made by a panel of judges. The elemental pool of statements in a Likert scale is not chosen (as in a Thurstone scale) to represent a spectrum of viewpoints ranging from one extreme to the other. Instead, the judges act as a pilot group, indicating their own response to each statement in a spectrum of categories ranging from **strongly agree** to **strongly disagree.**

After appraising each statement as being basically favorable or unfavorable to the phenomenon being measured, the investigator (rather than the judges) assigns scores so that each response is rated appropriately according to its favorable or unfavorable direction. If five categories are used in the judges' scale of elemental responses, the scores might be $-2, -1, 0, +1,$ and $+2.$

When the judges' pattern of responses is reviewed, the investigator uses a complex mathematical procedure, called *item analysis,* to eliminate elemental statements that do not show appropriate correlations in the internal analysis of scores. After these eliminations, the remaining statements presumably correlate well enough with one another to be regarded as reasonably homogeneous in demonstrating the phenomenon being measured. About 12 to 20 of these "good" items are then chosen as the constituent statements of a scale that reflects the scope of the phenomenon under assessment.

When the scale is subsequently administered, the respondent's scores for the individual items are added to form the output score. A Likert scale thus resembles an Apgar score, being formed as a *summation* of individual scores rather than representing a single distinctive point on a monotonic line. If everything has worked well, the summation process produces a clearly ordinal set of values for the scale. If things have worked extremely well, the scale may even approach the equi-interval characteristics of dimensional data.

9.2.4. GUTTMAN SCALES

Although Likert scales are easy to construct, the results do not have a consistently monotonic pattern. An output score of **0** can be obtained from two particular statements that the responder has designated as **0** and **0,** or as

+1 and −1, or as +2 and −2. Guttman's goal[76] was to produce a consistently monotonic scale, in which the contents of any single output category would hierarchically subsume any of the categories below it.

An example of such monotonicity was shown earlier for the ethnic prejudice index in Section 9.1.2. Another example of a monotonic subsuming-category scale is the following ordinal list of gradations for a person's ambulatory ability: **run over hurdles, jog, walk uphill, walk on level ground, ambulate indoors without help, ambulate indoors with help, unable to walk.** Someone who can accomplish any one of the tasks in this ordinal array can presumably accomplish all of the sequential tasks that succeed it.

Because of this monotonic or subsuming quality, the Guttman scale is sometimes called a *cumulative* scale, although *hierarchical* may be a clearer term. Its construction requires a complex mathematical procedure, called *scalogram analysis.* Because of the immense difficulty of getting a truly cumulative monotonic arrangement for multivariate data, Guttman scales are difficult to construct and have not become popular.

Figure 9.1 contains Venn diagrams showing basic goals in the three main psychosocial strategies for constructing output scales.

9.2.5. OTHER VARIATIONS

The theories used for psychosocial rating scales are presented in a vast literature, where interested readers can find descriptions of additional principles that can modify or supplant the basic "big three."[11,26,152] The modification process was used, for example, to construct an index of satisfaction with medical care. The investigators at first formed a Thurstone Scale, which was then discarded as unsatisfactory after several years of testing.[86] Preserving many of the original Thurstone items, the investigators next converted the index into a Likert scale, which was also later regarded as sub-optimal.[158] Keeping the basic Likert pattern, but using a modified "Scale Product" system of scoring developed by Eysenck and Crown,[35] the investigators then prepared the final scale used in their main research.[87] The results are discussed in Section 9.4.

9.3. **Theory of Evaluation**

In conventional forms of laboratory science, the evaluation of a measurement process has become a relatively traditional exercise called *quality control.* The results are checked for their *reproducibility* when the process is repeated and for their *accuracy* in approximating what is obtained by a reference or "gold standard" measurement.

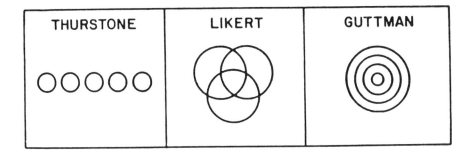

Figure 9.1. *Venn diagrams showing basic goals in the three main types of psychosocial scales.*

The Thurstone differential scale is intended to provide a single unique category from a group of linearly ranked choices that do not overlap. In this illustration, the respondent would choose one of the circles, thus identifying a single, unique location on the scale.

The Likert summation scale resembles a Boolean cluster. If each circle in this illustration represents a single category, the respondent can choose a location in the diagram that would score as 1, 2, or 3 categories. A score of 1 and a score of 2, however, can each be obtained in three different ways because of the overlap of the categories.

The Guttman cumulative scale, which is intended to produce a unique value, resembles a group of imbedded subsets, with each category encompassing the ones that lie beneath it. This subsuming arrangement creates the hierarchical monotonicity desired in the scale.

The attributes of reproducibility and accuracy are retained in the evaluation of psychosocial indexes, but several other attributes are also added, and the diverse entities are given a different set of names. The term *reliability* includes the idea of reproducibility, but it also refers to internal consistency or homogeneity of the components of an index. For example, the components of an index may each be reproducibly measured, but they may not fit together in a coherent manner. The term *validity* includes the idea of accuracy, but it also refers to the suitability of an index in performing its assigned task. Thus, we may have an accurate way of measuring the size of the pupil of the eye, but the measurement may not be a good index of anxiety.

The different methods used to identify and evaluate reliability and validity are a major part of theory in psychosocial indexes. The investigators have been challenged by a much more complex set of problems than the relatively simple demonstrations of reproducibility and accuracy for laboratory data in other forms of scientific research. The use of multiple component items and variables has added the extra challenge of dealing with their coherence or internal consistency. The development of new constructs when multiple variables are analytically aggregated produces the need for proving that the constructs are reasonable and effective. The application of individual indexes for different purposes creates the requirement for checking whether the same single index works equally well in diverse functional roles. The frequent absence of a gold standard for measurement entails the development of alternative techniques that substitute for an appraisal of accuracy.

In approaching these challenges, the investigators have developed an extensive set of concepts, methods, and vocabulary for delineating the particular ideas that become regarded as reliability and validity. The investigators have also developed and applied an extensive set of statistical procedures for converting the ideas into quantitative expressions. Because the diverse ideas and statistical procedures will receive detailed discussion later in Chapters 11 and 12, only one main point about them will be noted now. The words *reliability* and *validity* may evoke different qualitative concepts in the mind of a reader, but the concepts are not evaluated qualitatively in psychosocial theory. Whatever ideas are contained in those concepts are eventually transferred into a statistical format, and they are expressed with mathematical models that produce quantitative statistical coefficients.

The statistical methods of psychosocial theory have become one of the main ingredients of research and education in those fields. We are usually surprised to find medical clinicians who understand statistics, but we generally expect psychosocial scientists to be connoisseurs. Although very few physicians have tried to teach statistics or write books about it, psychosocial scientists (sometimes to the dismay of statisticians) regularly do such teaching, have written many textbooks on the subject, and have made major innovative contributions to statistical methods and scholarship.

The use of statistical methods—like the quest for dimensional data—has allowed psychosocial investigators to improve and harden the scientific quality of research concerned with the soft phenomena of human behavior. The obvious advantages of statistical methods, however, are accompanied by some important analytic and interpretive hazards. Analytically, ideas about reliability and validity undergo at least three main judgmental decisions before appearing as a quantitative statistical expression. The first decision involves the choice of the particular concepts that will be addressed by the model of a mathematical mechanism for appraising reliability or validity; the second involves the choice (and adequacy) of the mathematical model that performs the assigned task; and the third involves the choice of the particular group(s) of people whose data receive the mathematical analysis. All three of these soft judgmental decisions are fundamental issues in evaluating the hard data that emerge, but a focus on the quantitative results may sometimes distract the evaluator from giving adequate attention to the basic underlying qualitative appraisals.

In addition to the analytic hazard, the statistical methods also bring an interpretive hazard. If all three underlying judgments—about concepts, models, and groups—are satisfactory, the statistical coefficient can be received with confidence and can be interpreted as demonstrating what it purports to show for the particular aspects of reliability and validity that are under scrutiny. While concentrating on the intricacies of the chosen concepts, the mathematical mechanisms, and the selected groups, however, the evaluator may lose track of another basic scientific goal: sensibility. The diverse attributes that make an index sensible cannot be measured with statistical coefficients and must be appraised with qualitative judgment. The interpretive hazard of the statistical coefficients is that their impressive quantitative results for the goals of reliability and validity may distract the evaluator from thinking qualitatively about the sensibility that may be the most important goal of all.

Because sensibility is often the prime goal of clinimetric indexes, and because a theory has not been developed for the evaluation process, the next chapter is devoted to clinical methods for evaluating sensibility. As noted in previous comments and in that chapter, the goal of sensibility may sometimes compete for priority of emphasis against the reliability and validity that are the goals of standardization. If both sets of goals cannot be given prime emphasis, a conflict may occur. The investigators and collaborating consultants may or may not be aware of the conflict, but it is usually resolved at the beginning of the work when priorities of emphasis are chosen either inadvertently or with deliberate awareness and "informed consent."

If everything works out well afterward, the original choices of goals may not be recalled or reviewed. If things do not work out well, however, the investigators may conclude that fate was unkind, or that the research was too difficult to be done well, while overlooking the possible role of an unsatisfactory choice among the competing goals.

9.4. Example of a Problem Arising from Conflicting Goals

To illustrate the kind of problem that can arise from the conflict in clinical and psychosocial goals, I wanted an example of older rather than recent work, so that current controversies could be avoided. I also wanted an example of work done by outstanding investigators whom I greatly admire. The purpose was to ensure that the comments would not be construed as personal criticism, and to demonstrate that the conflicts can cause difficulty even for outstanding investigators.

Such an example is provided by the index of satisfaction with medical care, previously mentioned in Section 9.2.5. The index was developed for use in a study sponsored by a group of family physicians. They believed that patients receiving this type of medical care would be more satisfied with it than with the care given by internists or by other medical specialists. Trying to get documentary evidence for this belief, the family practitioners enlisted help from a group of academic investigators, based in a school of public health, who constructed an index "for the measurement of attitudes toward physicians and primary medical care."

The index was eventually applied to a "probability sample" of 1,713 adults in a midwestern community. Although the project was first described[86] in 1970, the final results were not reported until five years later.[87] The results of the satisfaction-with-care index, when correlated with the particular type of clinical practitioner who was used for primary medical care, showed that the "specialty of the regular physician" was *not* "associated with level of satisfaction."

The disappointing outcome of the study seems to have been accepted with equanimity by the professional organization of family physicians who sponsored the research, and the investigators who wrote the reports were kind to their sponsors. The reports emphasized the relationship between satisfaction with care and various demographic or socioeconomic features of the patients rather than with the specialty of the physicians. The results have not been highly publicized (despite the enticement they must have offered for specialists and other non–family physicians), and the index developed for measuring satisfaction with care has not come into general usage.

A review of the process with which this index was constructed and evaluated may reveal several problems as reasons why it has not been well accepted and why it did not obtain supporting evidence for the original hypothesis.

The index was developed with a classical psychosocial orientation, aimed at constructing a Thurstone scale. The three main "content areas" to be covered by the index were "professional competence, personal qualities, and cost/convenience." The investigators began with "a total of 300 statements with approximately 100 in each content area." After various types of editing, "149 statements remained with approximately 50 in each content area." From results obtained when these 149 statements were scored by a panel of carefully selected judges, the investigators then developed "two distinct scales, each containing 12 to 14 items from each of the three content areas." The dual scales were developed "to test for parallel form reliability" by noting the statistical correlation between "subsets of statements within each of the three content areas."

After this testing, the investigators selected "statements in a given content area ... from both scales." These statements were then "united to create three different scales, each of which contained two subsets of statements with comparable scores." The output scale derived in this manner contained 41 statements, which were then administered in a pilot survey to 254 residents of another city.

On reviewing the results, the investigators said that they "became aware of certain inadequacies of the scales." In particular, "the designation of items to each of the three content areas may not have been completely valid." For example, an item regarded as an indication of professional competence may have been interpreted as reflecting personal qualities; another item designated as "cost/convenience" may have been interpreted as a measure of professional competence. To deal with this problem, the authors asked a group of "39 experienced public health nurses" to reclassify the content areas of the statements in the index. The investigators also had the "distinct impression ... that respondents found the 'agree-disagree' alternatives uncomfortable."

Accordingly, the investigators revised their questionnaire to use "Likert-type response alternatives" and to remove a few old items and add new ones while retaining "judged scale values consistent with the Thurstone approach." In addition, the investigators developed a new scoring scheme for each item, based on "a modification of the Eysenck and Crown Scale Product method." The Eysenck-Crown strategy,[35] which is intended to do a better job than Thurstone or Likert scores in making "full use of the information available," attempts to create scores that "place a person's attitude on a straight line continuum from positive to negative affect."

The statements contained in this revised scale are shown in Figure 9.2, together with the scores (the "transformed scale value") for each statement and the direction (the "affect") in which each item was to be scored as positive or negative. The results of this new approach were reported as showing that the "Scale Product scores were consistently more reliable than scores computed using the Thurstone method of scoring." The investigators did not report any deliberate appraisal of the suitability or pertinence of the selected items as indexes of satisfaction with medical care; and their main emphasis was on the "reliability" of the scale in showing internal correlations among its various items and scores.

The investigators now believed that they had taken care of a major limitation in previous indexes of satisfaction: "the reliance on direct questions of unproven reliability and validity." With the new approach, the investigators hoped to eliminate the problems that often occur because "most respondents supply the socially acceptable answer and a quantitative attitudinal score for each respondent is not readily obtainable." This new version of the index was then applied to the group of 1,713 adults, who produced results that were so disastrous for the original hypothesis of the family physicians.

The investigators obviously used admirable diligence in carrying out the psychosocial goals of index development and in showing the high internal

Transformed Scale Value			Affect of Item
		I. Professional Competence	
2.26	1.	People do not know how many mistakes doctors really make.	Neg
3.32	2.	Today's doctors are better trained than ever before.	Pos
1.77	3.	Doctors rely on drugs and pills too much.	Neg
1.01	4.	Given a choice between using an old reliable drug and a new experimental one, many doctors will choose the new one.	Neg
1.96	5.	No two doctors will agree on what is wrong with a person.	Neg
2.85	6.	Doctors will not admit it when they do not know what is wrong with you.	Neg
1.14	7.	When doctors do not cure mildly ill patients, it is because the patients do not cooperate.	Pos
3.04	8.	Doctors will do everything they can to keep from making a mistake.	Pos
3.30	9.	Many doctors just do not know what they are doing.	Neg
.56	10.	Doctors spend more time trying to cure an illness you already have than preventing one from developing.	Neg
.21	11.	Doctors are put in the position of needing to know more than they possibly could.	Pos
1.92	12.	Even if a doctor cannot cure you right away, he can make you more comfortable.	Pos
2.59	13.	Doctors can help you both in health and in sickness.	Pos
1.38	14.	Doctors sometimes fail because patients do not call them in time.	Pos
		II. Personal Qualities	
1.21	1.	You cannot expect any one doctor to be perfect.	Pos
1.77	2.	Doctors make you feel like everything will be all right.	Pos
.70	3.	A doctor's job is to make people feel better.	Pos
1.63	4.	Too many doctors think you cannot understand the medical explanation of your illness, so they do not bother explaining.	Neg
2.52	5.	Doctors act like they are doing you a favor by treating you.	Neg
2.29	6.	A lot of doctors do not care whether or not they hurt you during the examination.	Neg
2.03	7.	Many doctors treat the disease but have no feeling for the patient.	Neg
1.04	8.	Doctors should be a little more friendly than they are.	Neg
2.34	9.	Most doctors let you talk out your problems.	Pos
2.13	10.	Doctors do their best to keep you from worrying.	Pos
3.68	11.	Doctors are devoted to their patients.	Pos
.08	12.	With so many patients to see, doctors cannot get to know them all.	Pos
3.11	13.	Most doctors have no feeling for their patients.	Neg
3.28	14.	Most doctors take a real interest in their patients.	Pos
		III. Cost/Convenience	
2.21	1.	Nowadays you really cannot get a doctor to come out during the night.	Neg
1.86	2.	You may have to wait a little, but you can always get a doctor.	Pos
1.93	3.	It is easier to go to the drugstore for medicine than to bother with a doctor.	Neg

(continued on next page)

Transformed Scale Value			Affect of Item
2.81	4.	The more money you have, the easier it is to see the doctor.	Neg
1.11	5.	A doctor has a right to charge what he does since he struggled for years to become a doctor.	Pos
2.96	6.	In an emergency, you can always get a doctor.	Pos
.04	7.	There just are not enough doctors to go around.	Pos
1.59	8.	Doctors try to have their offices and clinics in convenient locations.	Pos
1.42	9.	More and more doctors are refusing to make house calls.	Neg
.57	10.	People complain too much about how hard it is to see a doctor.	Pos
.90	11.	It is hard to get a quick appointment to see a doctor.	Neg
.39	12.	Doctors should have evening office hours for working people.	Neg
2.91	13.	Most doctors are willing to treat patients with low incomes.	Pos
3.63	14.	A doctor's main interest is in making as much money as he can.	Neg

Figure 9.2. Scale items in questionnaire for "Satisfaction with Health Care." The right-hand column shows the transformed scale value assigned to "agree" or "disagree" responses for each of the items cited in the middle column. Each of these responses is then cited as positive or negative, according to the affect of the item indicated in the right-hand column. For example, if someone agrees with the first statement, it has a value of −2.26.

Source: S. J. Zyzanski, B. S. Hulka, and J. C. Cassel, Scale for the Measurement of 'Satisfaction' with Medical Care: Modifications in Content, Format and Scoring, *Med. Care* 1974;12:611–20.

reliability of the scales. For clinical goals, however, the index seems unsatisfactory in features of sensibility that are often called "face validity" or "content validity." To discern those features, take a close look at the items listed in Figure 9.2. Do those items suitably represent the phenomena that the family physicians had in mind when trying to show the satisfaction of their patients?

Although different people will obviously have different opinions about what is "suitable" or "sensible," two characteristics of the 42 items listed in Figure 9.2 should evoke universal agreement. The first characteristic is that the items are stated in the general impersonal manner, discussed in Section 4.1, which has sometimes been used in psychosocial approaches. Despite the many merits of this policy, the statements do not invite the respondents to comment on their feelings about their own personal physician. The statements are aimed at beliefs held by the public about doctors in general. Consequently, the responses to those statements may reflect this general appraisal rather than the responders' individual feelings about their own doctors. The high "reliability" of the results may reflect the respondents' agreement in identifying this general consensus, although their own individual opinions have not been expressed.

A second prominent problem in the statements is their suitability for indicating satisfaction with care. Some of the statements seem to have little pertinence for determining a patient's satisfaction with an individual physician. Among such statements are the following (noted with their location in Figure 9.2):

I-2. Today's doctors are better trained than ever before.
I-13. Doctors can help you both in health and in sickness.
II-1. You cannot expect any one doctor to be perfect.
II-3. A doctor's job is to make people feel better.
II-12. With so many patients to see, doctors cannot get to know them all.
III-3. It is easier to go to the drugstore for medicine than to bother with a doctor.
III-10. People complain too much about how hard it is to see a doctor.

You may want to regard various other statements in the group of 42 as not being particularly pertinent to an individual patient's satisfaction with an individual doctor, but the seven just cited seem especially unsuitable.

It is entirely possible, of course, that a different index, with more personal orientation and more suitable contents, might also have been unsuccessful in showing the superior degrees of satisfaction anticipated by the family physicians. Nevertheless, because of the cited problems in face validity and content validity, the constructed index does not provide an adequate assessment of satisfaction with health care. Perhaps the main lesson to be learned from this project is not its information about "correlates of satisfaction and dissatisfaction with medical care," but an awareness of the profound difficulty that can arise when clinimetric goals in suitability of content are pursued with psychosociometric strategies that emphasize different goals.

Chapter 10

The Theory and Evaluation of Sensibility

In contrast to the well-defined principles that constitute theory for statistical and psychosocial activities in measurement, clinimetric indexes are usually developed without a formally established set of goals. Like many of the component variables that must be dissected from the clinician's intuition to form an index, the clinimetric goals exist but are also often intuitive. Clinicians know what they want, but often have difficulty expressing it with explicit stipulations.

Perhaps the main reason for this problem is that the clinical goals refer to issues in sensibility—an attribute that is difficult to define and even more difficult to quantify. An enormous amount of thought, work, and specification has gone into the theory with which standardization is often pursued as a goal of statistical and psychosocial indexes, but analogous attention has not been given to a theory of sensibility. It is not prominently cited either as a target to be sought when clinimetric indexes are constructed, or as an accomplishment to be checked when the indexes are evaluated.

The statistical and psychosocial goal of getting a standardized index is well identified by the theory that cites principles, formulas, and calculations for determining reliability (or reproducibility) and validity (or accuracy), but no analogous specifications have been provided for determining sensibility. The purpose of this chapter is to propose a set of specifications that can be used both as theory in constructing clinimetric indexes, and as principles in evaluation.

The chapter will begin with some brief definitions that are intended to distinguish *sensibility* from the two other attributes that are commonly cited as goals in measurement. The other two attributes—which will be called *consistency* and *validity*—receive extensive discussion in Chapters 11 and 12. They are mentioned here now mainly to indicate that they are *not* included in the scope of topics considered as part of sensibility.

10.1. The Vocabulary of 'Evaluation'

When we evaluate a particular index, how do we decide whether it is good or bad, satisfactory or unsatisfactory? What can we look at? What do we look at? What should we look at? Answers to these questions are needed when we appraise either a new index or an old one, and when we decide what index to use if several are available to describe the same phenomenon. For example, many different indexes have been developed to provide diagnostic criteria for myocardial infarction, to offer prognostic estimates for patients with chest pain, to classify the status of patients with cancer, and to rate the magnitude of such entities as anxiety, relief of pain, functional capacity in activities of daily living, and even quality of life. If we want to use an index for describing these phenomena, which index should we choose?

In laboratory work, the system of evaluation calls for measurements to be checked for their *reproducibility* when the process is repeated, and for their *accuracy* when the substance is measured with a standard reference procedure, or gold standard. Because these attributes cannot be checked in exactly the same way for most psychosocial indexes, and because various other attributes must also be checked, psychosocial investigators have created their own nomenclature for the activities. The same terms are also often applied in the evaluation of clinimetric indexes, although the vocabulary is often confusing. The two main ideas, to be discussed in the next two sections, refer to *consistency* (or "reliability") and *validity*.

10.1.1. CONSISTENCY

An important scientific attribute of a measuring system is its *consistency* in yielding the same result when the measurement process is repeated by the same method or observer (*intra-observer variability*) or by another observer (*inter-observer variability*). The term *consistency* seems much better than the psychosocial term *reliability* for describing this attribute. In general parlance, *reliability* carries a connotation of trustworthiness that may not be present if the same measurement yields the same results. A ruler that repeatedly measures 10 cm as 8 cm and a lunatic who repeatedly says he is Napoleon Bonaparte are both consistent, but neither is reliable. Among the alternative terms, *reproducibility* and *repeatability* have the disadvantage that they cannot be checked if the measurement process cannot be carried out again for exactly the same specimen or entity. Consequently, *consistency* seems to be the best name for this attribute.

In statistical parlance, the idea is often called *precision*. If repeated measurements of the same entity are all close to the same value, statisticians will refer to the measurement system as *precise*. In the mathematical model, a mean and standard deviation are determined for the set of repeated measurements, and a coefficient of variation is calculated as the quotient of the standard deviation divided by the mean. The lower the value of the coefficient of variation, the more precise is the method of measurement. This statistical usage of *precision,* however, is quite different from the scientific role of the same word. Scientists use *precision* for the amount of detail provided by a measurement system, not for reproducibility. For example, a method that can measure π as 3.14159 is more precise than a method that measures it as 3.1. A method that measures π as 5.82716354 is more precise than either of the two preceding methods, but the precise result is wrong.

To avoid the misleading connotation of *reliable,* the ambiguity of *precision,* and the problem of using and choosing between *reproducible* and *repeatable,* the word *consistent* will be preferred throughout this text.

10.1.2.   VALIDITY

Another important attribute of a measurement is *accuracy*. In scientific processes, this attribute is usually assessed by determining the agreement between the observed measurement and the result obtained with a standard reference system. Unfortunately, the idea of *accuracy* cannot always be applied to psychosocial or clinical indexes, because an unequivocal reference standard does not exist or cannot be obtained. We have no unique reference standard against which to compare ratings of anxiety, relief of pain, or functional capacity. When we establish criteria for the diagnosis of systemic lupus erythematosus, the criteria themselves become the reference standard, and we have no other external standard for judging them. We can see whether the results of the criteria agree with the diagnostic consensus of a panel of experts, but the process is not a test of accuracy. Similarly, when we examine a clinician's competence by noting answers to questions in a certification test, the answers can be rated as correct if they agree with the answers chosen by the certifying authorities, but the clinician's answers would not be regarded as accurate.

To avoid the problem of trying to evaluate attributes that cannot be tested for accuracy, psychosocial scientists have replaced the term *accuracy* with *validity,* and have used *validity* to refer to how well an index does its job. Unfortunately, because an index can do many jobs that are tested in many different ways, the word *validity* has been preceded by a diverse collection of terms that often tend to confuse rather than clarify the issue under consideration. Psychosocial scientists have developed at least 16 different words[123] as prefixes for *validity*. Among them are *face, content, construct, criterion-related, concurrent,* and *predictive.*

Some of these terms refer to attributes that can be appraised with statistical correlations and expressed quantitatively. Others (such as *face validity*) refer to qualitative attributes that are appraised with various forms of scientific common sense. To avoid introducing a new term, the word *validity* will be retained here for the various attributes (discussed further in Chapter 12) that can be assessed with quantitative statistical correlations.

The face validity and other *qualitative* attributes of an index, however, are often its most important features in clinimetrics, but their appraisal is often neglected because "common sense" is not easy to delineate. The commonsense attributes, however, are the things that clinicians evaluate as sensibility. The rest of this chapter contains an identification and specification of the qualitative attributes that can be catalogued under the general title of *sensibility.*

10.2. Sensibility in Clinical Indexes

The sensibility of a clinical index is appraised with what might be called "enlightened common sense," which is a mixture of ordinary common sense plus a reasonable knowledge of pathophysiology and clinical reality. The different attributes considered as part of *sensibility* were almost all discussed in previous chapters, but the attributes were dispersed in diverse places during the discussion. In this chapter, the attributes will be reassembled and cited in a single collection, where they can form a type of "checklist" for appraising sensibility. The topics under discussion are evaluated in a purely qualitative manner by a reviewer thinking about what the index contains and what it does. The issues that require quantitative evidence or other appraisals of specific data will be discussed when consistency and validity are considered in subsequent chapters.

The evaluation of sensibility can be divided into five major topics, some of which have many subdivisions. The main topics are briefly outlined here to prepare the reader for the more extensive discussion presented later.

1. *Purpose and Framework:* Before an index can be evaluated, we need to know what it is supposed to do. Does it identify a state, denote a change, predict an outcome, or offer a guideline? Why is the index needed? What void does it fill or what defect does it repair? In what kind of clinical situation is it applied? The answers to these questions about *clinical function, justification,*

and *applicability* are needed at both the beginning and the end of the evaluation. At the beginning, the evaluator needs this information to become oriented to what the index is doing. At the end, the information is needed for decisions about the success with which the index has achieved its stated purpose, superseded other analogous indexes, or become pertinent for the particular clinical problems to which it might be applied. For example, an index intended for use as a prognostic indicator cannot be regarded as successful unless it is accompanied by evidence of its prognostic efficacy. An index that requires data from a special test could not be used for routine clinical work if the test is not routinely performed. An index that is satisfactory for patients with insulin-dependent diabetes mellitus might not be satisfactory for diabetic patients who do not require insulin.

2. *Overt Format:* Regardless of how the contents have been chosen and put together, every index is expressed in an overt format. The format can be a single statement, for which a single response is elicited; or a long list of multiple statements or questions. Certain important features of sensibility can be discerned from a thoughtful review of the overt format, even if the reviewer knows little or nothing about the particular phenomenon at which the index is aimed. One such feature is *comprehensibility.* Do we understand what goes into the index and what emerges afterward? Another overt feature is *replicability.* Do the operating instructions clearly stipulate the ingredients that go into the index and the way they are put together? A third feature is the *suitability of the output scale.* Does it have an adequate scope, a logical pattern of ratings, and satisfactory capacity for discrimination?

3. *'Face Validity':* Although flaws in overt format can often be detected without any knowledge of the phenomenon to which the index is addressed, enlightened common sense is needed to appraise *face validity.* This term is often used for attributes of sensibility that can be discerned with judgments made from immediate appraisal of an index, without profound attention to its component parts. Among the things that can be noted in face validity are *focus of interpersonal exchange, choice of basic evidence, coherence of components,* and *suitable collaboration* of the person to whom the index is directed.

4. *'Content Validity':* The judgmental appraisal of the underlying components of an index is often called *content validity.* Like face validity, content validity cannot be evaluated with statistical methods because the decisions refer to qualitative features of suitability in the selection and aggregation of components. The following attributes are appraised as part of content validity: *omission of important variables; inclusion of unsuitable variables; weighting of variables; suitability of elemental scales; and quality of basic data.*

5. *Ease of Usage:* No matter how well an index is constructed, the process will be unappealing if it is too difficult to carry out. Consequently, the last main issue in sensibility refers to the amount of time, personnel, risks, and efforts involved in getting and organizing the data needed to express the results of the index.

In the sections that follow, each of these five main topics is discussed in greater detail. The 21 attributes that are noted in the titles of the subsections will become the features to be examined in a checklist for "sensibility."

10.3. **Purpose and Framework**

Every index has a purpose that is demonstrated by the clinical function it serves, and by the justification for its existence. Every index is also developed and applied within a particular framework of patients and clinical settings. These issues in function, justification, and applicability are evaluated to decide whether the index is needed or useful, how well it does its job, and how well it can be applied.

10.3.1. CLINICAL FUNCTION

As noted earlier, the four main functions of an index are to describe a state, denote a change, estimate a prognosis, or offer a guideline. The described state can be a noun, when the index shows the existence of a particular entity, or an adjective, delineating the severity, degree of magnitude, or qualitative characteristic of an existing condition. Changes in state can be noted from repeated use of a single-state index or from special transition indexes. When suitable additional information is appended, an index of state or change can produce a prognostic estimate or a managerial guideline. A single index might be used for one or more of these four functions.

When an index is first planned and reported, a statement about its functional role is essential. The statement lets the investigators know what to aim at when the index is constructed, and tells the evaluators what to look for in appraising its accomplishments. If the functional role of the index is not clearly specified, the subsequent evaluation is either impossible or an act of guesswork.

For example, after noting that no index has existed to express the severity of clinical illness in patients with cancer, an investigator could state that his purpose was to develop an index to fill that gap. Although denoting the general goal of the index, this statement of purpose would not be detailed enough to allow a suitable evaluation of how well the goal is accomplished.

How is the index of illness severity to be used? Is it going to act as a prognostic estimator? Will it express transitions between a pre-therapeutic and a post-therapeutic state? Is it supposed to demarcate sectors in the spectrum of disease so that the baseline distribution of different groups of patients can be compared before treatment? Unless these specific goals are explicitly stated, the investigator may not test the index in a manner that shows whether the goals are achieved. An index's accomplishments as a prognostic estimator, transition indicator, or baseline demarcator will require different types of data, but the necessary data may not be obtained.

A striking example of this problem occurred about a decade ago when an index of the "severity of renal disease" was proposed by a special committee.[21] The constituents of the index appear to have been carefully selected and assembled, but the results were presented without a specifically stated objective, and no explicit citations were offered for the way in which the index might be used. Since the index was not checked in a field trial, no data were appended to demonstrate what happened in actual usage. Despite the considerable work done by the original proponents, the index now appears to have been abandoned.

10.3.2. CLINICAL JUSTIFICATION

When a new index is reported, the investigator can be expected to state why it is needed, and why it is superior to analogous indexes that may already exist.

This type of justification is not always offered when a new laboratory measurement is developed. Thus, someone may arrange a new method of measuring serum molybdenum or urinary yttrium, because "it is there." Afterward, some useful role may be found for the measurements obtained and analyzed in a large series of patients. Clinimetric indexes, however, are almost never created in this manner. An investigator seldom goes to the trouble of constructing a new clinimetric index unless it is intended to do something, and to do it better than whatever was previously available.

The reasons for constructing an index and the rationale for its apparent superiority constitute the justification of the index. The justification is sometimes demonstrated (as discussed in Chapter 13) with documentary evidence obtained by comparing the results of the new and old indexes in a field trial, but usually the justification is simply a verbal account of what the investigator had in mind.

If the index offers a completely new expression for a phenomenon that was hitherto undescribed, the justification may be readily evident. If the new index, however, offers an alternative expression for something that already is cited with an old index, the investigator presumably had a special reason for creating the alternative expression. The evaluator can then see whether the desired goal was effectively achieved.

10.3.3. CLINICAL APPLICABILITY

The framework of an index is the medical (or non-medical) setting in which it was developed, and the particular kinds of people for whom it is pertinent. These distinctions will determine the clinical applicability of the index.

An evaluation of applicability involves attention to both the function and the framework of the index. In function, an index that was satisfactory for one functional role may not work well for another. For example, an index that is readily applicable for making a clinical diagnosis of the existence of angina pectoris may not adequately distinguish changes in the clinical severity of angina. Another index, which is excellently applied for identifying changes in status, may not be effective for predicting future outcomes. An index that is quite satisfactory for diagnosing coronary disease as an outcome event in the clinical course of originally healthy people may not work well when applied to diagnose coronary disease as the baseline state in a trial of therapy.

The framework of an index is particularly important for appraising its component variables and the spectrum of clinical subgroups to which it can be applied. For example, if an index is being used to diagnose coronary disease for patients admitted to a trial of therapy, the available data (and therefore, the component variables) will differ according to whether the therapeutic trial begins when the patient is admitted to or discharged from the hospital.

The framework is also important for showing the spectrum of clinical subgroups to which the index might be applied. A review of this spectrum will help demonstrate whether the index is too fine or too coarse for its clinical pertinence. For example, an index that pertains only to white men, ages 35 to 44, with "classical" angina pectoris and no accompanying co-morbidity, may focus on too fine a subgroup to have clinical value beyond that subgroup. Conversely, an index that refers only to patients with "classical angina pectoris" may be too coarse for clinical application because the clinical spectrum of "classical angina pectoris" is too heterogeneous. To make decisions for individual patients, clinicians may need further subgroup distinctions in the severity and co-morbidity of the angina.

The choice of subgroup distinctions is a taxonomic rather than clinimetric problem, arising not from the index itself, but from the way in which the index was developed, tested, and reported. Investigators who are aware of the pertinent clinical distinctions can arrange the reports accordingly, but in many instances, indexes are published without a citation of the additional taxonomic details. An index that seems satisfactory in its clinimetric construction may then be unsatisfactory for clinical application.

For example, a group of patients in TNM Stage III of a particular cancer may seem homogeneous because they share the same taxonomic classification, yet prognosis and therapy for the individual patients in Stage III may differ dramatically according to distinctions of clinical severity of the cancer and co-morbidity. When the results of a particular index (such as survival time or quality of life) are provided for all patients in Stage III, but not for subgroups of patients with different degrees of clinical severity and co-morbidity, the information may be satisfactory for a general statistical comparison of two treatments, but the results will not have the taxonomic pertinence needed for decisions in clinical practice.[47,52] For those decisions, the clinician would want to know the post-therapeutic results in appropriate clinical subgroups of patients, not just in the heterogeneous mixture assembled as **Stage III.**

Similarly, an index that classifies degrees of severity of congestive heart failure as **none, mild, moderate,** and **extreme** may be worthwhile for estimating prognosis in many patients with acute myocardial infarction, but may not be clinically cogent for predicting the outcome of the infarct in a 75-year-old man who has congestive failure together with a major arrhythmia and severe chronic lung disease.

The same type of problem occurs in statistical reports of the indexes used as diagnostic marker tests. No matter what type of mathematics is used for the calculations of sensitivity, specificity, likelihood ratios, or other statistical summaries, the results found in broadly defined groups of diseased and non-diseased patients are not taxonomically precise enough to indicate what would be found for patients in diverse parts of the associated clinical spectrums.[56]

Although few clinimetric indexes can be tested and reported with all of the possible details, the results in cogent clinical subgroups are essential to demonstrate the clinical applicability of the index.

10.4. **Overt Format**

In contrast to the clinical judgment needed to evaluate an index's pertinence for its purpose and framework, certain important attributes can be appraised, without any specific clinical knowledge, by someone who is familiar with three major challenges that pertain to any -metric activity. These challenges—which refer to the index's comprehensibility, replicability, and suitability of output scale—are appraised with principles discussed in the sections that follow.

10.4.1. COMPREHENSIBILITY

Comprehensibility, like beauty, is in the eye (and mind) of the beholder, and cannot be defined with a fixed set of rules. Nevertheless, four main principles that contribute to comprehensibility can be noted from observations of indexes that have become popular and useful. The principles can be cited under the titles of simplicity, oligovariability, transparency, and biologic connotation.

10.4.1.1. *Simplicity*

Simplicity, when appropriate, is always a virtue. It helps in understanding, remembering, and using whatever is being considered. The simplicity of an index is best discerned in the expression of the output scale. Thus, an additive index such as the Apgar score—which ranges from **0** to **10** and which requires a simple sum of five component scores, each having the values of **0, 1,** or **2**—will be relatively easy to use and to remember. The simplicity of usage and recall will vanish if an index, such as the Norris score for prognosis of myocardial infarction, is obtained with the formula $3.9x_1 + 2.8x_2 + 10x_3 + 1.5x_4 + 3.3x_5 + 0.4x_6$, as described earlier in Section 3.4.2.1. This process requires the addition of variables having a wide range of dimensional values, some of which are transformed into diverse ordinal scales, and all of which receive different weighting coefficients before the addition is carried out.

A numerical rating or score is usually easier to comprehend and deal with than an array of adjectives. For this reason, many clinical rating scales are expressed in numbers such as **0, 1+, 2+, 3+, 4+**, rather than in verbal expressions such as **none, slight, moderate, substantial,** and **extreme.** Simplicity of expression is also a reason for the frequency with which global rating scales and binary scales of existence (e.g., **yes/no, present/absent,** or **normal/abnormal**) are used in clinical activities.

Although a simple output scale has major importance, simplicity is also desirable, when possible, in the ingredients of the index. For example, as noted in Section 3.2, an index is simpler to deal with if all its component elements are clearly identified than otherwise, and if the original expressions of data have avoided conversion into some of the unusual or esoteric transformations noted in Section 3.6.

10.4.1.2. *Oligovariability*

Another way to keep things simple is to limit the number of different variables contained in the index. If the Apgar Score had included ten variables, rather than five, the appeal of the index might have been sharply reduced, and it might never have achieved its current popularity. Similarly, the clustered categories of the TNM staging system are relatively easy to remember and understand as **I, II**, and **III**. They are derived from component variables that refer to the tumor's size, primary-site characteristics, involvement of regional lymph nodes, and involvement of distant sites. A more complex staging system, which still creates clusters, may have the prognostic advantages of adding important additional variables, such as symptom severity and co-morbidity, but the contents of the index will be initially more difficult to comprehend except in the extreme stages, where all the "good" or all the "bad" features are clustered together.

On the other hand, the advantages of a simple output scale and few component variables may not compensate for the disadvantages produced if the scale does not function effectively. Thus, despite desirable simplicity and oligovariability, the existing TNM staging systems have many defects as prognostic indexes for patients with cancer.[59] The improvements will require the inclusion of more variables and the additional complexity they will bring.

10.4.1.3. *Transparency*

The type of transparency discussed in Section 5.3.2 obviously depends on the number of variables contained in the index. The fewer the number of component variables, the more easily a user can see through the output scale to determine the constituents of a particular index rating.

Another determinant of transparency, however, is the number of categories in the rating scale used for each component variable. For example, because each of the five variables of the Apgar score can be expressed in one of the three ratings of **0, 1**, or **2,** the total number of possible underlying combinations is $3 \times 3 \times 3 \times 3 \times 3 = 243$. Some other scale, having only three variables rather than five, may initially seem more transparent than the Apgar score, but the scale will become more "opaque" if each of those three variables has a rating scale of **0, 1, 2, ..., 5, 6.** With seven values available for each of the three variables, the total number of possible underlying combinations will be $7 \times 7 \times 7 = 343$. The three-variable scale will therefore have more possible combinations than the Apgar score.

A third feature that affects the transparency of a scale is the variation of weighting coefficients (or of individual rating scales) in an additive score. Thus, in the Apgar score and in the scale cited in the previous paragraph, each component variable had the same individual rating scale (either **0** to **2,** or **0** to **6**) and the same weighting coefficient (which was 1 in both indexes). In an index such as the Norris Score, however, the use of a regression formula such as $3.9x_1+2.8x_2+10x_3+\ldots$ makes the index doubly opaque. It has different weights as well as different individual rating scales for each variable.

10.4.1.4. *Biologic Connotation*

The principle of biologic connotation is cited here because it can help the comprehensibility of an index. The basic idea will be cited again later, when we consider the biologic coherence of components as an attribute of face validity.

Although indexes expressed as combinations of numerical scores often have the virtue of simplicity, the result may be difficult to understand not only because of problems in transparency, but also because the score cannot be readily associated with a biologic connotation. Conversely, the categorical contents of a Boolean cluster may be more complex to express than the arithmetical result of a mathematical score, but a categorical cluster is often much easier to explain.

For example, consider a previously discussed index for the three clinical manifestations of *inspiratory rates, peripheral edema,* and *distended neck veins.* In an additive score, each of these manifestations might be rated **0** if absent and **1** if present. If all three manifestations were present, their combination would receive a score of **3.** This score would be clear and appropriate, but it would not evoke the same immediate clinical recognition and understanding as the explicatory name, **congestive heart failure,** which might be given to a clustered category containing all three elements.

The biologic coherence of the components—as noted later in Section 10.5.3—can be helpful in evaluating as well as understanding the contents of an index. For example, the cluster category, **pregnant man,** is understood and produces no problems in comprehension, but the category is biologically impossible.

10.4.2. REPLICABILITY

The replicability of an index refers to the clarity and thoroughness of the directions that are provided for its usage. When an index is used by someone other than its creator, can those other people easily discern what to do and how to do it?

The principle of replicability differs from the principle of consistency (or reproducibility). Replicability is determined as a qualitative judgment, derived from reading the operational directions that accompany the index. Consistency is determined as a quantitative statistical result, derived from field trials that examine variability among the same or different users of the index. These studies of variability, which are discussed in the next chapter, require the collection of a group of entities and observers, application of the index to each entity by each observer, and an appropriate statistical analysis of agreements and disagreements. Replicability, however, can be appraised from a direct examination of the index itself.

10.4.2.1. *Clarity of Instructions*

To appraise replicability, we look at the operational description of the index and ask whether all the ingredients have been adequately stipulated. If we cannot determine exactly what goes into the index and how everything is put together, the index will not have high replicability regardless of how good the statistics may seem for quantitative studies of variability.

As discussed earlier in Section 3.2, problems of replicability usually arise when the basic ingredients and aggregation of the index have not been suitably specified. The operating details may show the ratings to be given to such entities as **hypotension** or **pulmonary edema,** and the way in which the ratings are combined for the output scale, but no specifications may have been given to indicate exactly what is meant by **hypotension** or by **pulmonary edema.** Other problems in replicability occur when the index is expressed in a global scale, without explicit criteria for demarcating the ratings that are cited in the scale. In the absence of such explicit criteria, a global scale may have many of the advantages discussed in Chapter 7, but the individual single-state ratings given by different people may not be standardized.

A different aspect of replicability arises in self-administered indexes. The problem here is to be sure that the user, rather than the evaluator, understands the instructions. A clinician evaluating the instructions may think they are pellucidly clear, but many patients may be confused or uncertain. The challenge for the creator (and evaluators) of an index is to place themselves in the position of a wide variety of users, to decide how those users will react to the instructions, and to clarify whatever needs clarification.

Other issues in replicability involve clear instructions and standardization for any mechanical devices or other procedures that accompany the use of the index. For example, the account of an exercise stress test may have good stipulations for when to stop the test and how to give an appropriate rating if the patient develops chest pain, but the mechanical device employed in the test may not be well described or well standardized. Some of the many difficulties in the diagnostic accuracy of exercise stress tests can be ascribed to this problem. Originally, the patients went up and down portable tiers of two or three steps; later they pedaled on a stationary bicycle; now they walk on a moving treadmill. If the operation of the treadmill is not standardized, the process will be difficult to replicate.

Another aspect of replicability, as noted in Chapter 6, refers to the role of effort and support, and also to the choice of a patient's threshold symptoms or maximum tolerance when magnitude is cited for a performed task. If those distinctions are not suitably managed, the reported "magnitude" can vary substantially without any real changes having occurred.

10.4.2.2. *Unbiased Examining*

Because the attitudes and expectations of the person who conducts an examination or interview can obviously affect its results, double-blind techniques are commonly used in clinical trials of therapy. The same precautions are often necessary, but often omitted, when an examiner asks the questions, does the testing, or gives the ratings for a clinimetric index. For example, an interviewer can easily become biased by a knowledge of the research hypothesis, or by attributes of the interviewed person's gender, appearance, socioeconomic status, or style of speech. Unless suitable objectivity is sought in appropriate circumstances, the results of the index may be untrustworthy as well as non-replicable.

10.4.3. SUITABILITY OF OUTPUT SCALE

At least two important attributes of suitability can be discerned from a simple inspection of the output scale, without any deeper judgmental attention to its components. These attributes are the comprehensiveness and discrimination of the scale.

10.4.3.1. *Comprehensiveness*

The comprehensiveness of an output scale was previously discussed in Sections 5.1.1 through 5.1.4. The scale should have an exhaustive scope of categories; the categories should be mutually exclusive; they should be exhaustively inclusive in providing locations for all the possible combinations of input data; and the scale should have realistic values. When an index contains combinations of categories from input variables that are monotonic, either the resulting scale should be unequivocally monotonic or the pattern of ratings should allow places for irregular mixtures of categories, as discussed in Section 5.4.2.

10.4.3.2. *Discrimination*

An output scale should allow easy discrimination of the desired distinctions for comparing single states of different people or different states of the same person.

A scale that is too coarse does not contain enough categories to provide the desired distinctions. For example, if clinical competence is rated in a **pass/fail** grading scale, the results may be quite satisfactory for many decisions; but they may not allow an effective ranking of candidates for the development of a class standing. Conversely, a scale that is too fine contains more categories than can be used for effective or consistent choices. Thus, if the clinical loudness of cardiac murmurs is to be graded on a scale of **0, 1, 2, . . . , 98, 99, 100,** the scale will be extremely difficult to use because it requires a nicety of discrimination that cannot be achieved with clinical auscultation.

Coarseness of scales is a particularly common problem in clinimetric indexes that have relatively few categories. For example, the **I, II,** and **III** categories of the TNM staging system for cancer can be used effectively to describe the general state of patients with cancer, but the identification is too coarse for many clinical decisions in patient care. Because any one of the three stages will contain a heterogeneous spectrum of patients, the results noted for prognosis or therapy in a particular stage will be difficult to apply to single patients and difficult to compare in groups of patients.

The converse problem—excessive discrimination—may make certain scales difficult or unattractive to use. The problem is particularly pertinent for indexes whose output is expressed as a profile of subscales. For example, the *TNM Profile Index* for cancer is cited with such profile ratings as **T0N2M1, T3N1M0, T4N0M2,** etc. The profile ratings contain a high descriptive content, but the number of possible categories is so great that the indexes are seldom used for comparing spectrums of patients or for evaluating prognosis and therapy. To be more effectively applied, the many different ratings of the *TNM Profile Indexes* are clustered into three main ordinal categories, which are labeled as the **I, II,** and **III** groups of TNM Stages. An excessive number of categories in the profile scale of the index of severity of renal disease, discussed in Section 10.3.1, may have been another factor contributing to that scale's lack of acceptance in the clinical community.

The problem of comparison becomes particularly striking when a coarse single-state scale is used to determine *changes* in the same person. For example, a patient's clinical condition can be dramatically improved from miserably moribund to asymptomatically ambulatory while the patient's cancer remains in Stage **III.** If the **I, II, III** staging system is the only method of measurement for determining change, the improvement cannot be recorded.

The measurement of change can also be impeded if the index has too many variables (as discussed in Section 5.2.3) or has an unsuitable focus. An example of the latter problem was shown in the previously discussed (Section 9.4) psychosocial index of satisfaction with health care. If an individual clinician, after changing his professional style of behavior, wanted to see whether the change made his patients more satisfied, the index would probably not show the effects. The index calls for patients to rate the behavioral style of doctors in general rather than the performance of their particular doctor.

To avoid the difficulties arising from excessive variables, inadequate focus, or excessively coarse scales, investigators can use separate indexes of transition, which are intended (see Section 5.2.4.2) to deal directly with expressions of change. The transition data can supplement or sometimes replace the dyadic ratings of change that are achieved from comparisons of two single-state readings.

10.5. 'Face Validity'

In most psychosocial discussions of the formulation and evaluation of indexes, face validity is regularly mentioned, acknowledged as important, given a brief bow, and then ignored thereafter as the discourse proceeds to other forms of validity. Although the value of face validity is obviously appreciated, it receives relatively little direct attention because it cannot be measured statistically and it is difficult to define judgmentally.

Nevertheless, particularly for indexes that are intended to reflect the complex observations and dissected intuitions of clinical experience, face validity is often the most important attribute of the index. If aimed at the wrong thing or put together in the wrong way, the index will lack sensibility and will be unsatisfactory no matter how many statistical accolades are acquired in subsequent field trials.

The appraisal of face validity is often contemplated with a type of global approach in which the evaluator makes decisions using implicit but unspecified variables and criteria. The subsections that follow are intended to dissect this global intuition about face validity into four explicitly specified attributes that can receive individual appraisals. The attributes refer to the focus of interpersonal exchange, choice of basic evidence, coherence of components, and attention to suitable collaboration.

10.5.1. FOCUS OF INTERPERSONAL EXCHANGE

Whenever an index is applied, an interpersonal exchange occurs between the respondent and the examiner (or the questions). As previously discussed

(Section 4.1.3), the focus of this exchange may be off target if the quest for objectivity leads to asking the wrong kind of questions or getting an inappropriate form of personal data. The problem was illustrated when inquiries about satisfaction with medical care were phrased in an impersonal way that would elicit responses about general public opinion rather than individual personal attitudes. The problem can also occur when self-administered questions, designed to be answered without any assistance, are misunderstood and channeled into directions that were not intended in the original plans.

To evaluate suitability of interpersonal exchange, the reviewer can determine whether the information being sought is supposed to reflect personal attributes or beliefs of the interviewed person. If so, is the information being solicited in a manner that will evoke an accurate, candid account of those attributes or beliefs?

10.5.2. FOCUS OF BASIC EVIDENCE

The focus of basic evidence in an index may be unsuitably displaced in several ways that were discussed in Section 4.1. The actual phenomenon being described may be altered from a soft entity, such as chest pain, to a hard entity, such as an electrocardiographic finding. The scope of the phenomenon may be constricted from the desired information about functional capacity in daily life to data about performance in a laboratory exercise test. The intrinsic attributes of a phenomenon, such as the characteristics and location of a pain, may be replaced by an extrinsic account of its functional impact on the patient; and the severity of an illness, as manifested by its consequences in the patient, may be replaced by evidence of its impact on therapeutic or other decisions made by a clinician.

These various substitutions and displacements may be appropriate and justified in many circumstances, but unsuitable and unwarranted in others. The decision about suitability will depend on both the particular phenomenon described by the index and the specific purpose of the index. If the purpose of the index and the kind of evidence it contains are in agreement, the result will be suitable. Otherwise, the index may have an inappropriate focus in its basic evidence.

Attention to this type of suitability is part of the reasoning used when an investigator decides what kind of basic evidence to assemble as candidate components for the index. Additional forms of suitability arise, as described later, when decisions are made about which candidate variables to retain and which ones to omit or exclude. Because the results of these decisions are difficult or impossible to evaluate quantitatively, the appraisal of their sensibility is almost always an act of qualitative judgment.

When we appraise the focus of basic evidence, the main concern of face validity is that the entire index is unsuitable, being directed at the wrong target. For example, an index that contains only tests for esoteric information about sporting events or movie stars would seem overtly unsuitable for assessing intelligence, clinical competence, or quality of life. In the appraisal of content validity, as discussed in Section 10.6, the main concern is that the index, although aimed at the right target, has an impaired suitability because of inappropriate omissions or inclusions. Thus, an index that deals with cognitive information and challenges in rational reasoning, but that lacks attention to imagination and creativity, would have impaired suitability for measuring intelligence. Quality of life would not be well appraised by an index that emphasizes physical function while ignoring a person's emotional function and individual goals in life. Since these sources of unsuitable contents will be discussed under *content validity,* the two other attributes to be included under *face validity* refer to the coherence of the components and the attention given to the collaboration of the user.

10.5.3. BIOLOGIC COHERENCE OF COMPONENTS

As discussed in Section 5.3.1.1, coherence refers to the way things go or fit together, according to their mutual rather than individual suitabilities. Coherence can be evaluated for the group of variables that are aggregated in an index to form a mathematical score, or for the particular categories that are joined into individual Boolean clusters. Thus, the values of age and height may both be suitable components of an index, but does it seem sensible to add their two values together to form a single score? If selected categories of age and height have been joined to form a scale of clusters such as **tall young people, short old people,** and **all others,** do the categories of tallness and youngness fit together in a sensible manner? Do shortness and oldness seem appropriately joined for whatever purpose the index is to be used?

The issue of coherence becomes an important part of face validity when multiple variables have been arbitrarily aggregated into a single composite index. The aggregation may not create major problems if the index identifies a single state—such as the Apgar Score for a newborn baby or a set of diagnostic criteria for a disease. The aggregation may be difficult, however, if the composite index is used repeatedly to show changes in state. For example, composite indexes for the state of patients with rheumatoid arthritis[111,143] or with inflammatory bowel disease[157] contain an array of many different variables. They refer to specific symptoms of the disease, pathophysiologic derangements, abnormalities in laboratory tests, and functional disabilities. Although each of these components has distinct importance, the meaning of their aggregated score is difficult to interpret clinically, and changes in a patient's score from one occasion to the next are even more difficult to interpret. For this reason, the aggregated scores of these multi-composite indexes have sometimes been used for appraisals in therapeutic trials, but have lacked the face validity that would make them accepted in clinical practice.

10.5.4. ATTENTION TO PERSONAL COLLABORATION

The last main feature of face validity is the attention given to the collaboration of the person to whom the index applies. As discussed in Section 6.3, the role of collaboration—which is somewhat analogous to the role of compliance or adherence in the maintenance of therapy—has been overlooked in most clinimetric indexes concerned with a patient's performance of a task. The index itself seems to have face validity because it is usually aimed in a reasonable direction at a reasonable target, but the main problem is in the validity of the results. Unless suitable attention has been given to the patient's motivation, effort, and support in performing the task, a rating for magnitude of task will be uninterpretable as well as nonreplicable.

The absence of such attention impairs the validity of many task-performance indexes that have been used in both clinical and epidemiologic research. The problem is particularly cogent when the indexes are used to denote post-therapeutic change, because the contributions of therapy often cannot be differentiated from the effects of alterations in motivation, effort, or support.

10.6. 'Content Validity'

In face validity, we look at the suitability of overt features of the index's formulation, aggregation, and application. In content validity, we dig more deeply to evaluate the suitability of the component parts. The evaluation deals with the omission of important variables, the inclusion of unsuitable variables, the weighting of variables, the elemental scales, and the quality of basic data.

10.6.1. IMPORTANT OMISSIONS

The things that have been left out of an index are sometimes more important than what has been included. The problem was illustrated earlier with the rejection of content validity for a written examination alone as a measure of a clinician's competence, and for an IQ test that contains no attention to imagination or creativity.

A striking clinical example of the omission of important variables occurs in the prognostic staging of cancer. Although perceptive clinicians have known for many years that *severity of illness* is an important predictor of outcome for patients with cancer (or with many other diseases), this variable has been almost universally omitted in prognostic indexes. The main reason for the omission has been the absence of a clinimetric index for classifying severity of illness. In recent years, the importance of illness severity has been acknowledged after such unexpected discoveries as the demonstration that an index of performance status in patients with cancer was prognostically more cogent than the conventional morphologic contents of the TNM staging system.[131]

After contemplating what variables seem clinically important and suitable, and after noting what has been included in an index, a reviewer can determine what has been omitted. There can be several reasons for the omissions:

1. The variable may have been tested and found to be unimportant; if so, the investigators have presumably shown the evidence.
2. The variable may have been tested and found to correlate closely with another variable that was used instead. For example, *hemoglobin value* may be omitted from an index that uses *hematocrit value.*
3. The variable may have been considered and discarded, without testing, because some other variable was chosen as a preferable substitute. Thus, *performance status* may have been regarded either as a suitable surrogate for *severity of illness,* or as a better index.
4. The variable may have been considered but left unanalyzed because it does not have its own index and scale for clinimetric citation. (This is the probable reason *severity of illness* is omitted.)
5. The importance of the variable may not have been recognized.

In the last three situations, the main problem in the composite index is the absence of suitable methods for including and testing potentially important component variables. To improve the quality of the index, the first step would be to provide suitable clinimetric development of the absent components.

The omission of important components is particularly striking in indexes that are used for establishing diagnostic status, describing outcomes, and estimating prognosis. In diagnostic status indexes, for example, the co-morbid ailments that can exist in addition to the main disease are almost never mentioned, even though the concomitant occurrence of such ailments is a common clinical event.[41] The absence of citations for co-morbidity may then greatly impair the clinical pertinence of the diagnostic index, because its performance has not been identified in the appropriate subgroups of co-morbid patients.[56]

In outcome indexes, the description of post-therapeutic events has usually been confined to such hard data as survival and dimensional changes in tumor size or laboratory data, with minimal or no attention given to the quality of life of the treated patients. In prognostic indexes, the absence of soft data is particularly troublesome. Many soft clinical features that are cogent predictors of a patient's subsequent course are regularly omitted from staging systems or other indexes of prognosis. Among the cogent soft data are severity of illness, patterns of symptoms, duration and progression of illness, and severity of co-morbidity.

10.6.2. INAPPROPRIATE INCLUSIONS

The suitability of the included components can usually be promptly discerned by noting their appropriateness for the stated or inferred purpose of the index. Although appropriateness can sometimes be evaluated by common sense alone, a background of clinical knowledge will often be required. For example, a person with no clinical training could immediately discern that **stool frequency** seems suitable and **urinary frequency** seems unsuitable as components of an index of *inflammatory bowel disease*. A person with no clinical background, however, might not promptly recognize that **swelling of ankles** is an appropriate component for an index of *congestive heart failure*, but not for an index of *headache severity*.

Decisions about suitability of components can also depend on nuances of the exact role to be played by the index. For example, as an ingredient in an index concerned with angina pectoris, *magnitude of task required to evoke chest pain* might not be particularly useful if the index is employed for making the diagnosis of coronary heart disease, but the ingredient would be appropriate if the index is devoted to transitions in the severity of angina.

Other aspects of suitability may require arbitrary clinical judgments about which not all evaluators will agree. For example, suppose a specific task, such as *placement of both hands simultaneously behind neck*, is included as a component of an *index of functional capacity*. Some clinicians will claim that this task is an appropriate feature of functional capacity. Others will argue that mobility of the upper limbs can be better appraised with some other challenge.

For these reasons, the components included in an index are probably best rated as clearly suitable, clearly unsuitable, or equivocally suitable. The evaluator can usually promptly decide whether a particular component is clearly suitable or unsuitable. Components that are equivocally suitable can be rated on the basis of the stated justifications for their inclusion.

In the discussion thus far, the emphasis was on the suitability of individual attributes of the included variables. A separate issue in suitability of included components arises when a single-status index contains a summary value for a variable that has been measured at successive points in time. For example, to denote the pre-treatment value of blood pressure, we might have many readings available, based on blood pressure measurements made at many times before onset of treatment. The single value to be used as the pre-treatment status can be calculated as an average of all the available values, as the modal reading, as the single most recent reading, or in some other fashion. The appropriateness of the decision will depend on the pattern of the available values both for individual persons and for the total group of people under study.

10.6.3. WEIGHTING OF COMPONENTS

Another distinctive attribute, which is analogous to coherence, is the sensibility of the relative weights (or importance) assigned to different components of an index. The judgments used in the weighting process may be performed differently by different people, particularly when decisions are required for utility or human values. For example, although dyspnea and peripheral edema can each be components of an index of congestive heart failure, many clinicians (or patients) may regard having dyspnea as worse than having edema, or vice versa.

The weighting of components is particularly cogent when composite indexes are constructed for complex phenomena such as functional disability, quality of life, health status, or satisfaction with medical care. Because the importance of each of the component variables may be rated differently by individual patients and clinicians, striking disagreements can often arise about the sensibility of the decisions. A professional athlete may be much more distressed by an impairment in visual than in auditory function; a professional writer may be more distressed by an impairment in vision than in locomotion; and some patients might gladly exchange impaired sexual function for impaired locomotion, or vice versa. The importance of a patient's preference in these matters was discussed earlier in Section 6.4.3. In fact, when important individual preferences are ignored, the index may have an unsuitable basic focus, and the problem may be a matter of face validity rather than content validity.

The problem of weightings becomes particularly prominent when the weights are chosen by a mathematical model rather than by judgmental mechanisms. As noted in Chapter 8, the weights that emerge from the statistical analysis can be affected by certain caprices of the mathematical model, by the particular collection of data, or by the operational parameters of the data processing. With different models and operational parameters,[46,155] the coefficients for certain variables in the same set of data can receive strikingly different weights or even different directions (in positive or negative signs). The evaluation of sensibility for the weights assigned to different component variables is therefore particularly important when the assignment has been made without the use of clinical judgment.

10.6.4. SATISFACTORY ELEMENTAL SCALES

Even if an index has all the basic components and weightings that make its contents seem suitable, the component variables may not have been expressed in a suitable manner. The scales of the elemental component variables—rather than the output scale of the aggregated index—may be unsatisfactory for any of the reasons that were previously cited in Section 5.1. Some of the elemental scales may lack a suitable neutral category, such as **uncertain** or **indeterminate,** that may be needed for diagnostic or other decisions that cannot always be expressed in a definite **yes** or **no** direction. Other elemental scales may be too coarse (such as **old** and **young** for *age*) or too fine (such as **1, 2, 3,..., 98, 99, 100** for *clinical loudness of murmur*) to permit adequate discrimination of the described phenomenon. Yet other scales may also be defective in exhaustive scope or use of mutually exclusive categories.

Perhaps the greatest problem in elemental scales, however, is their nonexistence. The absence of an appropriate scale for citation is probably the main reason, as discussed previously, for the omission of important component variables in clinical indexes. A variable may be omitted because it lacks a scale or because an existing informal scale (such as **1+, 2+, 3+, 4+**) is regarded as too soft for formal usage. The problem can easily be solved by hardening the soft scale with stipulations and criteria for a standardized demarcation of the categories, but the challenge is often neglected or rejected. Consequently, a problem that often impairs the preparation of a suitable composite index is the absence of a suitable elemental scale for some of the necessary components.

10.6.5. QUALITY OF BASIC DATA

Finally, even if everything else seems satisfactory, the evaluator may have scientific reservations about the process of observation and reporting that converted the basic phenomenon into the entries noted on the elemental rating scales. At this level of evaluation, the issue refers to scientific quality of the basic data, rather than to the construction of a clinimetric index.

In ordinary laboratory activities, the basic data consist of a direct measurement of a single variable, such as cholesterol or glucose. In clinimetric activities, however, the basic data can be direct primary observations, such as *diastolic blood pressure 77 mm Hg.,* or secondary designations, such as *petechia,* that represent an interpretation of an unexpressed primary observation of the skin. The primary observation for a petechia, if recorded, might be a statement such as "erythematous zone, blanching with pressure, surrounding a non-blanching darker-red central zone."

For the paraclinical data obtained from laboratory tests, a set of strict methods and standards has been established to maintain quality control when an observational process transforms a particular entity, such as a specimen of serum, into such primary data as **cholesterol = 325 mg/dl,** and when primary data are converted into a secondary interpretation such as **hypercholesterolemia.** For clinical data obtained during history taking, physical examination, and clinical reasoning, however, an analogous set of methods and standards has not been established for the processes that convert observed clinical entities into data.[38] The development of such methods and standards is an important aspect of clinimetric activities, but is beyond the scope of the discussion here. The clinimetric evaluations have begun with the assumption that the raw data exist and have a satisfactory quality, regardless of whether the starting points are primary observations or secondary interpretations.

10.7. **Ease of Usage**

The importance of this last-cited attribute is obvious. It refers to the amount of time, the concomitant efforts and hazards, and the type of personnel needed to collect the information used in the index. No matter how well an index has been constructed, tested, and reported, it cannot be satisfactory if it is too time-consuming, hazardous, or costly to apply. If the acquisition of data for the index requires special devices, such as the display of a computer program at a video terminal, or if the data processing involves other special techniques, such as a programmable electronic hand calculator, the characteristics and complexity of these technologic adjuncts should be identified and recognized.

Since most clinimetric indexes involve phenomena determined by history taking, physical examination, or clinical reasoning, there will seldom be any risks to be considered from invasive technologic procedures. Occasionally, however, when the index is constructed as a mixture of clinical and paraclinical data, the associated risks of getting the paraclinical information should also be noted.

Another feature of ease of usage is acceptability by the people to whom the index is applied. For example, if the index contains questions about sexual, personal, familial, economic, or other information that individual persons may be reluctant to discuss with a relative stranger, and if the questions are not phrased in a suitably discreet manner, the index may fail because it does not receive adequate cooperation.

A more obvious but separate problem in usage is the operating procedure itself. The questionnaire may be too long, the wording may be cumbersome, or the instructions may be unclear. Difficulties of this type should ordinarily be discovered and remedied during the early pilot tests of the index, but certain indexes may sometimes enter general usage without having received such tests.

10.8. Synopsis and Conclusions

The 21 principles that have just been cited can be used, somewhat like a review of systems in a patient's physical examination, as theory for identifying the sensibility of a clinimetric index. The principles are summarized and recapitulated in Table 10.1 on page 166.

Although these features of sensibility are often the most important things that determine the clinical success or failure of an index, they are often ignored when formal evaluations are conducted. The most likely reason for this neglect is that no mathematical techniques have been developed to provide numerical expressions for purpose and frame of reference, comprehensibility, replicability, suitability of scale, face validity, content validity, and ease of usage. Unlike consistency and the types of validity that are discussed in the next two chapters, the diverse attributes of sensibility require purely judgmental appraisals and cannot be expressed in statistical terms.

In an era of quantophrenic attention to mathematical expressions, many clinical investigators are reluctant to rely on judgmental strategies, even when the judgments refer to such fundamental distinctions as sensibility. The main reason for devoting an entire chapter to these judgmental appraisals is to indicate their priority in clinimetric importance, and to suggest ways of dissecting the judgments into specific decisions that can be identified with scientific precision and clarity.

If an index is not sensible, it does not warrant all the subsequent efforts used to demonstrate its consistency, criterion validity, and construct validity. If the index successfully passes the screening test provided by these fundamental judgments about sensibility, however, the remaining attributes can then be evaluated, as discussed in the next two chapters, with the appropriate qualitative and quantitative statistical techniques.

Table 10.1. Features to Be Considered in Appraising the Sensibility of an Index

Overt format	Purpose and framework	Clinical functions Clinical justification Clinical applicability
	Comprehensibility	Simplicity Oligovariability Transparency Biologic connotation
	Replicability	Clarity of instructions Unbiased examining
	Suitability of scale	Comprehensiveness Discrimination
	Face validity	Focus of interpersonal exchange Focus of basic evidence Biologic coherence of components Attention to personal collaboration
	Content validity	Important omissions Inappropriate inclusions Weighting of components Satisfactory elemental scales Quality of basic data
	Ease of usage	

Chapter 11

The Evaluation of Consistency

After an index has been developed, its scientific quality must be "validated." The validation process is complex, because it is aimed at many different attributes. The process is also confusing for clinical readers, because it often involves unfamiliar statistical expressions and because the attributes themselves are given familiar names that are used in unfamiliar or ambiguous ways.

In psychosocial vocabulary, the main activities of statistical validation are called *reliability* and *validity*. As noted briefly in previous chapters, however, *reliability* is not as good a term as *consistency*, and the idea can refer to two different things: the external "observer variability" with which an index is used and the internal inter-relationship of the component elements of the index. *Validity* can refer to at least four different ideas, which have been designated with names such as *face validity, content validity, criterion validity*, and *construct validity*.

For clinimetric purposes, validation often begins with the qualitative attributes of *sensibility*, which cannot be calculated statistically and which were identified and discussed in Chapter 10. Although the idea of *sensibility* does not have a specific name in psychosocial vocabulary, the attributes of sensibility include concepts that are often called *face validity* and *content validity*.

For subsequent activities in validation, the main goals are to determine the consistency (or reliability) of the index and its criterion validity and construct validity. Although the results are usually expressed statistically, the main principles involve an understanding of what is being evaluated and why. The principles will be discussed in this chapter for *consistency* and in Chapter 12 for *criterion validity* and *construct validity*.

167

11.1.   **The Basic "External" Concept of Consistency**

The term *consistency,* for reasons discussed in Section 10.1.1, is a preferable substitute for *reliability.* Regardless of which word is used, however, it can include two different ideas. The familiar idea refers to the "external" observer variability with which an index is applied on different occasions by the same user or by other users. The other idea, which is relatively unfamiliar to clinicians, refers to the "internal" inter-relationship of the component elements of the index. The internal distinctions will be discussed later in Section 11.5. The rest of this section is devoted to the traditional external concept of consistency.

An index has external consistency if it yields similar results when repeatedly applied to the same entity. This type of consistency might be tested by seeing what emerges when the same patients are rated again by the same clinician or by some other user of the index. When reapplied by the same person, the index is tested for *intra-observer variability;* when reapplied by some other person, the test shows *inter-observer variability.* If the repeated results have satisfactory agreement, they are regarded as consistent.

11.1.1.   SOURCES AND NOMENCLATURE OF INCONSISTENCY

Inconsistent results in repeated use of an index can arise from three sources. First, the entity under examination may change from one examination to the next. The particular substance that is being measured in serum may be unstable, or a patient's clinical condition may be altered between the two or more sets of successive observations. Second, the procedure itself may have its own intrinsic sources of variation. A chemical reagent applied during the measurement process may be unstable, or the instructions given for using a questionnaire or some other written format may be so vague, ambiguous, or unclear that the user is confused or uncertain about what to do. Third, the persons who apply the procedure may have their own variability when they use it. Thus, at least three different sources of variability can produce disagreements in repeated results.

The nomenclature used for labeling these three sources of variability is not standardized. The first source arises from variations in the particular entity—ranging from a specimen of dead tissue to an intact living person—that constitutes the input to the observational process. The term *input variability* seems better than *entity variability* as a title for this problem.

Many different names have been used for the second source of disagreements. It is sometimes called *method variability,* in reference to the different technical methods used for laboratory measurements, or *instrument variability,* in reference to the questionnaires or other structured formats that are the "instruments" used in collecting data for many indexes. Since the term *method* can be ambiguous (because it comprises both an apparatus and a user), and since many clinimetric indexes do not involve the application of a specific data instrument, the preferred title here will be *procedure variability.*

The third source of disagreement is usually called *observer variability*—a term that is also ambiguous, because it often refers to the results of the entire process rather than to the distinctive contribution of the user. This ambiguity can be eliminated by designating the third source as *user variability.*

With this convention in nomenclature, the three individual sources of disagreement can be called *input variability, procedure variability,* and *user variability.* The results of the entire process, without regard to individual components, can be appraised as *observer variability.* These terms, although perhaps not ideal for the appraisal of mensurational variability and quality control in laboratory work, seem less unsatisfactory than the alternative candidates for designating what happens when clinimetric indexes are appraised for external consistency.

11.1.2. THE SCIENTIFIC IMPORTANCE OF CONSISTENCY

Most persons thinking about the qualities that make data scientific would say that the information should be hard, but the attributes of hardness are seldom defined. When pressed to identify those attributes, individual persons may mention such features as accuracy, objectivity, dimensionality, and preservability. The information is *accurate* if the measurement obtained with a particular procedure closely agrees with the result obtained with a reference or standard procedure. The information is *objective* if the measurement is free of the various prejudices that may occur in human observers. The measurement is *dimensional* if it is expressed not in words, categories, or arbitrary ratings, but in a standardized scale of numerical values that have the equi-interval attributes discussed in Section 3.1.1.2. The mensuration process has *preservability* if the input entity—such as a specimen of serum, a piece of tissue, or a radiologic image—can be saved for reexamination at a later date.

Although often regarded as essential elements of hard data, none of these four attributes is a necessary feature of scientific information. The clouds, air currents, atmospheric pressures, humidity, and other input entities of meteorology cannot be preserved for reexamination, yet meteorologic data are usually accepted as scientific. The microtubules, mitochondria, and other entities seen with an electron microscope are described mainly with words rather than dimensional numbers, and the descriptions are produced subjectively by a human observer. Yet electron-microscopic data are usually accepted as scientific. Furthermore, a great many observations regarded as scientific data cannot be checked for accuracy because a universally accepted reference standard does not exist for the procedure. Among such observations are the histopathologic diagnoses made by a pathologist, the chromosomal abnormalities identified by a geneticist, and the infrastructural phenomena described by an electron microscopist.

Once we recognize that hardness of data does not require demonstrations of accuracy, objective observations, dimensional expressions, or preservable basic entities, we can concentrate on the prime requirement of scientific information: consistency. No matter how the observations are made and described, the data will have scientific quality if the results of the observational process can be consistently reproduced by the same or another observer.

If consistency is achieved, accuracy can readily be attained by the establishment of an appropriate reference standard. The standard may come from a process that produces an objective dimensional measurement of a preservable entity; it can be the opinion of a selected authority; or it can be derived from consensual agreement of a group of authorities. For example, a neophyte's interpretation of a histopathologic specimen is often regarded as accurate (or correct) if it is confirmed by the professor of pathology.

The role of consensual agreement in producing arbitrary standards of accuracy is often overlooked when scientists think about the qualities of hard data. Yet every one of the basic measurements of science—the duration of an hour, the length of a meter, the weight of a kilogram, and the volume of a liter—was created arbitrarily by a consensus of authorities. What allows these basic measurements to be scientific is not the accompanying standards of accuracy, but the ability to make the measurements in a consistent, reproducible manner. If the measurement process were not consistent, its accuracy could not be determined and might not be worth evaluating.

Realizing the paramount importance of consistency as the sine qua non of a scientific process of mensuration, we can turn our attention to the way consistency is achieved and later to the way it is evaluated.

11.1.3. ACHIEVEMENT OF CONSISTENCY

In the mensurational activities of a chemistry laboratory, each type of measurement is carried out according to a thoroughly stipulated operational process. Most clinicians, who themselves today seldom do such things as measuring serum glucose or counting white blood cells, have forgotten (or not learned) about the many pages of descriptive detail that are required to give adequate directions for these procedures. A suitable account of directions will describe all the many steps that must be taken to calibrate the equipment, prepare the reagents, handle the specimens, begin the process, carry out the intermediate operations, and observe the results.

Although equally necessary to produce the raw data and to do the subsequent conversions that create a clinimetric index, these detailed directions are seldom prepared or made available for clinimetric indexes. As discussed throughout Section 3.2, the stipulations may be missing for every level of the construction of an index, ranging from demarcation of the output scale to specification of the elemental ingredients.

There are many reasons for the omissions. In the preceptorial methods of clinical instruction, medical students and house staff are usually taught to do these procedures by observing their performance directly rather than by reading detailed accounts of the process. Even if detailed guidelines were available for observing the specific elements of the patient's history and physical examination that yield the raw data, too many things would have to be read. Even if time were available to do all the reading, the expenditure of the time might not be regarded as worthwhile because alternative types of information, obtained with various technologic methods, are usually regarded as more important, and often are more appealing because of their higher scientific quality. Even when the raw clinical data have reasonably good scientific quality, the process of converting the information into an index may receive minimal scientific attention.

As a result of these and other features of the state of the art in clinical education, a self-fulfilling prophecy has occurred for clinimetric activities. The information is often regarded as scientifically worthless because it is soft, and it remains soft because efforts are not made to harden it. The solution to this problem can begin as modern students and clinicians recognize the crucial importance of clinical data and clinimetric indexes. Once we realize again that such clinimetric entities as a patient's pattern of discomfort, functional status, and quality of life are often more cogent in clinical care than diverse technologic measurements, and that the information is hard in sensibility, we can start to improve its soft consistency.

Just as acts of research were responsible for developing the technologic procedures that produce modern forms of scientific data, scientific improvements in old forms of clinical data will also begin with investigative activities. After suitable research is done to improve the clinical data and indexes, and after the value of the improved information is perceived, the improved clinical procedures that produce the information can be absorbed into clinical education and routine care. During the research activities, many items of routine history taking and physical examination may be reappraised and found to have low value. Like old laboratory tests that are no longer pertinent or useful, this information may then be discarded or allowed to remain soft. The job of making clinimetric improvements will thereby be eased because it can focus on a smaller, more manageable number of entities that are emphasized not for tradition alone, but for their cogent sensibility and demonstrated value in patient care.

Although the consistency of a measurement process is usually determined with the "field trials" discussed later on, two important contributions to consistency occur before the field trials begin. The first contribution comes from the operational instructions and criteria that are developed when the index is originally constructed. The second contribution takes place when these instructions and criteria are tested (and improved) in pilot studies conducted before the field trials begin. These two activities will be discussed, respectively, in Sections 11.2 and 11.3.

11.2. The Role of Operational Instructions and Criteria

Just as a cook needs a recipe to prepare something new or unfamiliar, a person who is going to use an index must be given a suitable set of directions. If variations occur in the product that emerges when the recipe is used by different cooks, the differences might be due to the personal culinary vicissitudes of the cooks, but another source of inconsistency may be inadequacies in the recipe itself. A group of cooks whose culinary behavior is similar enough to produce exactly the same thing with a well-specified recipe might have great variations in the product if the recipe is ambiguous or confusing.

In applying a particular clinimetric index in a particular clinical situation, the user goes through a three-phase procedure. The user first observes whatever entity (patient, specimen, film, etc.) is the input to the process. In the second phase, the user converts those observations into raw data. In the third step, the data are converted into a designated category of the output scale. Although variability can occur, as discussed earlier, in the input entity and in the user's personal style of activity, our concern now is with variability in the mechanisms used for performing the three phases of this procedure.

The first phase, for reasons discussed earlier in Section 10.6.5, is beyond the scope of this dissertation. The particular processes that clinicians use during history taking, physical examination, and other acts of observation are obviously important and often paramount, but the activities are too complex for further discussion here. Methods of improving the scientific quality of these basic observational activities have been extensively described elsewhere.[38,53] Besides, in many clinimetric activities—particularly those conducted with patients' medical records and other sources of archival information—the observational process may have been performed, and its results recorded, by someone other than the user of the clinimetric index.

The second and third phases of the procedure are more inherently clinimetric. The second phase involves operational specifications for converting raw data into the particular variables, categories, or other ingredients that enter the construction of the index. These specifications, which might be called *ingredient criteria,* lead to the replicability discussed in Section 10.4.2 and earlier throughout Section 3.2. After these basic ingredients are delineated in phase two, they are converted, in phase three, to the category that emerges in the output scale of the index. The instructions for performing this phase can be called *conversion criteria.* They will be defective if the categories of the output scale are not clearly demarcated, if the output scale does not have a comprehensive scope, or if the output scale does not have adequate discrimination.

For example, the ingredient criteria will be unsatisfactory if the user is not told what level of blood pressure to designate as **hypotension** when hypotension is cited as a basic element in the index. The conversion criteria will have inadequate scope if no category is provided for citing the rating of a patient who has both hypotension and pulmonary edema. The conversion criteria will also have inadequate discrimination if they contain a category for citing both hypotension and pulmonary edema, but if the category is too coarse to allow the user to show distinctive improvements that may have occurred in either hypotension or pulmonary edema (or both) while a patient continues to have both manifestations.

Any of these (or other) defects in the operational specifications of ingredient criteria or conversion criteria can lead to variability in use of the index because the user will be uncertain about what to do. For example, a user who wanted to show that a patient's state had changed, but who could not show the change by assigning the "correct" rating offered in the scale of an index, might try using an incorrect rating that would show a change—thereby achieving sensibility while producing inconsistency. In this manner, a patient who is markedly improved but still bedridden might be erroneously designated as **ambulatory with substantial help** if the user of the scale had no category other than the repetition of **bedridden** with which to try to express the improvement.

Although often disregarded during the attention given to the statistical results of field trials, the operational details and criteria provided for an index are the prime determinants of its replicability, comprehensiveness, and discrimination. These sources of procedure variability must be evaluated with careful qualitative judgments; and they are often more important than input variability or user variability in contributing to the composite attribute that is evaluated as *observer variability.*

11.3. **The Role of Pilot Studies**

The person who creates an index almost always tries it out in various ways before the index is used in a formally reported research project. These try-outs, which are usually given the more dignified title of *pilot studies,* can be done in several ways. In the customary activities, the creator of the index will get collaborating colleagues to apply it to various patients. After seeing what sort of results emerge, how the results differ among different users and different patients, and how well the process is received by both users and patients, the creator of the index may then modify it. The modification will usually improve the contents, aggregation, instructions, criteria, or other arrangements of the index's construction and operational specifications. After these changes, a second round of pilot studies may be conducted, followed by another set of improvements. The process may then be reiterated until the construction and procedural criteria seem optimal.

At this point the index may be regarded as ready for application in formal research. The formal research may be either a field trial, intended to provide quantitative assessments of observer variability, or an actual investigation in which the index is used as one of many sources of data in the research. Thus, after pilot studies of a new index for rating the clinical severity of dyspnea, the investigators could do a formal test of its observer variability[118] and could also use the index directly in a randomized trial[119] comparing the effects of therapeutic agents in patients with chronic pulmonary disease or other sources of dyspnea.

In the -metrics of psychosocial research, a formal test of observer variability is almost always carried out and reported before the index is used in specific research projects. In clinimetric work, however, this formal test is often omitted, because the clinician and the psychosocial scientist may have different goals. Seeking sensibility as a prime virtue, appraising it during the informal pilot studies, and persuaded by the pilot results, the clinimetrician may be satisfied by the informal evidence showing that the index has suitable replicability, comprehensiveness, discrimination, and other appropriate virtues. The clinician may then decide to avoid "wasting time" with formal studies of observer variability, and may proceed directly to the specific research for which the index was developed.

Since the pilot studies were performed in an informal manner, they may be reported either with minuscule descriptions or not at all. Consequently, when the index first appears in its research application, an evaluator who tries to check the scientific background of the index may then be dismayed to find no quantitative demonstrations and no adequate qualitative accounts of its consistency. This mode of development has been commonplace for most of the clinimetric indexes in use today. Almost all the particularly well-known clinimetric indexes—such as Apgar Scores, TNM Stages, New York Heart Association Functional Classifications, and Glasgow Coma ratings—were developed and published without reports of pilot studies and without field trials of observer variability. In recent years, for example, field trials of observer variability were not done for a pictorial index of infant physical appearance, developed by Kramer et al.[106], and for other indexes, developed by my colleagues and me, for severity of illness,[50] co-morbidity,[41,45,48] and auxometry[13] in patients with cancer, for auscultatory diagnosis of rheumatic valvular disease,[37] and for changes in cardiac functional status.[49]

In these and many other situations, clinical investigators aiming at sensibility as a prime goal of the mensuration process may have believed that the sensible value of the index would better be demonstrated by its accomplishments in specific research than by relatively sterile tests of its observer variability. Wanting to show that the index works well enough to be clinically worthwhile, the investigators therefore went directly to research that would show that value. Subsequent investigators, persuaded of the index's sensibility but uncertain about its scientific quality, may then later conduct field trials of observer variability. In many instances, however, the index seems so sensible and useful (like Apgar Scores or TNM Stages) that it is promptly incorporated into clinical practice and becomes widely disseminated without any field trials having been done.

This distinction should be borne in mind when the scientific quality of clinical indexes receives critical appraisal. The things noted during the unreported pilot studies, together with the reported evidence of the index's sensible value in pragmatic clinical research, may not fully justify the absence of statistical tests of consistency, but may substantially mitigate the magnitude (or effects) of the scientific flaws.

A different, converse type of problem arises when a field trial is conducted, as discussed in the next section, before an index has been suitably evaluated and modified in pilot studies. This situation may occur if the investigators rely mainly on statistical coefficients—rather than on judgmental appraisals and on the stepwise assessments and improvements attained with small pilot studies—to indicate the scientific quality of an index. The main difficulty in this type of premature field testing is that the results may be greatly misleading. An index with a high statistical coefficient for consistency may have low sensibility; and an index that could easily become highly useful if given the appropriate pre-trial modifications may be dismissed because of a low statistical score in the field trial.

11.4. **The Role of Field Trials**

The name *field trial* refers to an organized formal study of the performance of a particular procedure in the actual circumstances for which it is proposed. The "field" can range from a community in which household interviews are conducted, to a hospital or other medical setting used for clinical activities. The trial can be intended to study observer variability, diverse types of validity, or both.

The design of these trials—an important scientific challenge that seldom receives as much attention as the statistical results—will be discussed in Chapter 13. The main point for consideration now is the frequent absence of field trials of observer variability for clinimetric indexes. If the trials are regarded as the sine qua non of scientific measurement, indexes lacking such trials will be scientifically unacceptable. Is this harsh verdict always deserved if an index has not received formal field trials of consistency?

One answer to this question was suggested earlier in Section 11.3. Consistency may have been checked and found adequate in pilot studies that were never formally reported. A second answer is that the demands for testing certain types of consistency may be inappropriate, because the process may be too difficult or impossible to do. For example, because we cannot schedule the delivery of babies and because newborn babies often change their condition rapidly, studies of observer variability are not feasible for the Apgar score. We could check the variability among observers who are present at each delivery, but we would have great difficulty in assembling the same group of observers for a series of different deliveries. Complete checks of inter-observer variability would also be unfeasible for procedures such as bronchoscopy or various types of endoscopy whose repetition may involve substantial discomfort for the patients. We could get the examiners to make their observations after the "scope" has been previously inserted,[18] but the patients would be too uncomfortable if each observer repeated the entire procedure from the start.

For a different set of reasons, we may not be able to test *intra*-observer variability in circumstances where clinicians can remember what they said previously if the second test is repeated too soon after the first. A delay of the second test, waiting to give the clinician a chance to forget what was noted previously, will be pertinent only if the condition of the patient is stable enough to be unchanged during the interval. Because of this problem, many clinimetric indexes are checked for inter-observer but not for intra-observer variability. Intra-observer—as well as inter-observer—variability can readily be tested, however, if the clinical user works with a set of recorded data, rather than a living patient, or with specimens (such as smears, tracings, films, etc.) that do not change between examinations.

A different explanation for the neglect of field trials is the entrenched medical tradition of *not* checking the consistency of basic data that are expressed subjectively. Observer variability is seldom tested by epidemiologists for information about exposures to suspected noxious agents, by clinicians for data about symptoms and physical signs, by radiologists for the interpretation of images, and by pathologists for designations of cytology and histopathology. If consistency is not regarded as important enough to be tested for basic data, it cannot be expected to attain importance for the combinations of basic data that appear in a composite index.

Perhaps the most common reason for a lack of field trials, however, is the apparent value of the information. Because the value of a new psychosocial index may not always be dramatically apparent, a demonstration of "reliability" is one of the main ways of getting potential users to accept the index as meritorious. Although the demonstration of consistency may be a necessary part of the persuasion that a new psychosocial scale has improved the measurement of a particular attribute, no persuasion may have been required for many clinical observations and for the results produced by histopathology, cytology, radiography, scintigraphy, or computed tomography. Since the medical information may be immediately regarded as valuable, the medical index can become accepted on the basis of face validity and content validity without any studies of observer variability. A new medical index can thus become widespread and commonly used before being subjected to any tests that might demonstrate its inconsistency.

Because of the different traditions in the medical and psychosocial domains, the two types of indexes thereby become produced with a striking paradox. Many psychosocial indexes that have high consistency may have dubious value, and many clinical indexes that have high value may have dubious consistency.

11.5. Additional Concepts of "Internal" Consistency

In everything discussed so far in this chapter, the basic idea of *consistency* referred to variability in external use of the index. Two additional concepts of internal consistency, however, are regularly considered by psychosocial scientists when they evaluate the total consistency (or reliability) of an index. The issues usually arise when an index is formed as the sum of scores for a large series of individual items, such as the plethora of questions asked in a written examination given to certify clinical competence, or the many individual items rated in the satisfaction-with-care index discussed at the end of Chapter 9. For these types of multiple-item indexes, the many individual items can be appraised for the consistency of their inter-relationships with one another.

These inter-relationships can be considered for two different attributes. One of these, which might be called *performance consistency,* refers to the performance of the individual items contained in different parts of the index or in repetition of the index by the same user. The issue here is not the external variability of the users, but the internal variability of the items contained in the index. A second attribute, which can be called *internal homogeneity,* refers to the coherence of the items in their intercorrelation with one another. These two additional types of consistency are discussed in the subsections that follow.

11.5.1. PERFORMANCE CONSISTENCY

Suppose we develop an index of clinical competence as the total score obtained by a candidate who answers a set of 200 questions in a licensure examination. If the total process performs consistently, and if we randomly divide the 200 questions into two groups of 100 questions each, we would expect the candidate to receive roughly similar scores for each half of the questions. This type of appraisal for the performance consistency of an index is called *split-half reliability.* It is statistically expressed as the correlation coefficient between the ranks of the scores of a set of candidates in a randomly chosen first-half set of questions and the corresponding ranks in the second set.

A somewhat different way of testing consistency in performance is called *test-retest reliability.* In this situation, the basic focus of the individual questions is maintained, but the questions themselves are altered to produce a different, second examination. For example, if the first examination contains three questions about movie stars, four questions about sporting events, and five questions about enzyme reactions, the second examination would contain a similar number of questions about the same topics, except that the questions would refer to a different set of movie stars, sporting events, and enzyme reactions. The same candidates would take both examinations, and a close correlation of their performance in the two examinations would be regarded as good evidence of test-retest reliability.

A different test-retest procedure is somewhat analogous to split-half reliability. For the first test, the candidate answers a random sample of half of all the questions. For the second test, the candidate answers the remaining half of the questions. (Regardless of whether the process involves new questions or a randomly chosen batch of previous questions, test-retest reliability requires an examination of two different versions of the same index. If exactly the same index is used on both occasions, the investigation deals not with performance of the index, but with observer variability in consistency of the users.)

In the psychometric analyses of formal examinations for clinical or other forms of competence, the same set of examination questions is seldom repeated for the same set of candidates because they will probably remember many of the first questions and look up the results afterward. A different version of the same type of questions can be constructed, however, for analyses of test-retest reliability. Because these different versions are not easy to develop, many psychometric analyses depend on split-half rather than test-retest reliability. Occasionally, however, a few examination questions that were used in one year may be repeated in a subsequent year. The results of these repeated tests—if the two groups of candidates are reasonably similar—can then be compared for test-retest reliability of the individual questions.

Because relatively few clinimetric indexes have been constructed in a multiple-item format, these issues in performance consistency are relatively unfamiliar to most clinical readers. Nevertheless, as indexes with multiple items have been used increasingly to describe complex phenomena such as functional disability and quality of life, statistics for split-half reliability and test-retest reliability have begun to appear in clinical literature.

11.5.2. INTERNAL HOMOGENEITY

In Section 5.3.1, we considered two approaches for showing the biometric coherence of the components of an index. The *bio-* approach relied on judgmental evaluation of the sensibility with which the components fit together. The *-metric* approach depended on a statistical demonstration of similar results in the data when each component was related to an external variable.

A different -metric strategy for evaluating coherence is commonly used in psychosocial indexes, but does not employ an external variable. In this strategy, the data are statistically analyzed for the way in which the components relate to one another. Thus, in the first -metric approach, we might examine the survival rate associated with individual items—A, B, C, and D. In the second approach, we would examine the way that items A, B, C, and D correlate with one another.

The inter-correlation of variables or component items is a useful way of checking the psychosocial goal of forming a unidimensional index. If the individual variables (or items) seem to correlate well or fit together closely, or if each pair of components has roughly equal correlations, the components may be regarded as being relatively homogeneous. They would then presumably measure the same thing, and would therefore produce an essentially unidimensional index.

The statistical mechanism used to check these correlations is a calculation of *Cronbach's alpha.*[25] (When the items are expressed in binary form, such as **yes/no** or **true/false,** the calculated result is called the *Kuder-Richardson coefficient, Formula 20.*)[108] Cronbach's alpha (or its Kuder-Richardson analog) is a coefficient of correlation, representing a weighted average of the interrelationships that exist when data for each component of the index are correlated with every other component. Like a coefficient of simple squared correlation for two variables, the values of Cronbach's alpha can range from **0** to **1.** Unlike the relatively low values found for many simple correlations, Cronbach's alpha is often quite high. Values are considered "good" if > 0.8 and "excellent" if > 0.9.

To illustrate the process, suppose we wanted to develop an index of erythematosity for blood, using measurements of hemoglobin, hematocrit, red blood count, reticulocyte count, and white blood count as possible component variables in the index. When applied to a large group of patients, the five components might not have a particularly high level of inter-correlation, as shown by Cronbach's alpha. A factor analysis, however, might show that hemoglobin, hematocrit, and red blood count seem to go together closely, whereas reticulocyte count and white blood count are separate factors. We might therefore eliminate reticulocyte and white blood count as components, and we would construct the index of erythematosity from only the first three variables (hemoglobin, hematocrit, and red blood count). An index containing only those three variables might have an extremely high value for Cronbach's alpha, thus suggesting that the three variables are homogeneous and are probably all measuring the same phenomenon. (You will be declared out of order if you now complain that the index will also have a high redundancy because its three elements are often synonymous. Had you wanted to think about scientific sensibility rather than statistical associations, you should have raised doubts earlier about the purpose and function of an "index of erythematosity.")

Cronbach's alpha is almost never calculated for clinimetric indexes because they are often constructed—like the Apgar score or TNM stages—as a deliberate composite of multiple variables that have different individual roles. As long as each component variable makes a distinctive contribution to the index, clinicians are willing to include that variable and to accept some of the subsequent problems that occur for unidimensionality, transparency, and monotonicity of patterns when multiple variables are aggregated.

If the composite result is used to identify the total aggregate of a particular condition, a clinician will want all of the important distinctions to be included in the composite expression. On the other hand, if certain variables are so closely related (such as hemoglobin and hematocrit) that one can often be substituted for the other, one of these variables might be eliminated because it does not make a distinctive contribution to the composite index. Thus, if heart rate, respiratory rate, color, tone, and reflex responses were closely correlated with one another in the Apgar score, a clinician might want to eliminate some of these variables from the index, rather than including all of them.

The apparent redundancy of closely correlated variables is also often deliberately avoided when clinimetric indexes are constructed with mathematical models, rather than with the type of judgment that led to the Apgar score. In such mathematical procedures as stepwise regression (discussed in Chapter 8), variables will be eliminated if they do not make sufficiently distinctive contributions to the total index. In psychosocial indexes, however, redundancy may be deliberately sought as a mechanism for achieving a reasonable degree of homogeneity from a group of multiple items. The psychosocial goal is aided by the method used for calculation of Cronbach's alpha. For example, if an index contains 3 items that have pairwise correlations of 0.3, Cronbach's alpha will be 0.56. If the index contains 20 items that have pairwise correlations of 0.3, Cronbach's alpha will rise to 0.90. Because an increased number of inter-correlated items may be "rewarded" by rising values of Cronbach's alpha, psychosocial scientists are statistically encouraged to enlarge the number of items in an index, but clinical investigators—working with different goals—may want to shorten the number of items, particularly by eliminating those that seem redundant.

From time to time, questions about internal homogeneity may arise for the components of a clinical index. For example, suppose we have found an aggregate of variables that act as an index for predicting survival. The external statistical coherence of the variables is easily appraised when each variable is examined separately for its univariate relationship to survival. The biologic coherence of the aggregated multiple variables, however, may be difficult to understand or check with any of the principles described earlier for sensibility. Consequently, as a possible substitute for the judgmental appraisal of internal *biologic* coherence for the variables, Cronbach's alpha may be calculated to show their internal *statistical* coherence.

11.6. Statistical Expressions of Consistency

Unlike sensibility, which can be evaluated qualitatively from thoughtful appraisal of the index itself, consistency is evaluated quantitatively from data produced in actual use of the index. The field trial that produces the data is designed according to the type of consistency (intra-observer, inter-observer, split-half reliability, etc.) under evaluation; and the suitable planning of these field trials is particularly important if the data themselves are to be scientifically acceptable for further statistical analysis. As noted later in Chapter 13, the statistical results of a field trial are often received and interpreted as the sole issue in evaluation, without adequate attention to the scientific quality of the trial itself. Since those problems will be discussed in Chapter 13, the rest of this chapter is concerned with the statistical methods used to express measurements of consistency.

Since issues in performance consistency and internal homogeneity were described in Sections 11.5.1 and 11.5.2, the discussion now will be concerned with the statistical measurement of the basic type of consistency that is called observer variability.

In the usual field trial of observer variability, the group of entities selected as input for the trial each receives two (or more) observations. For studies of intra-observer variability, each set of observations is made by the same observer on different occasions. For inter-observer variability, each set of observations is made by a different observer. The agreement between the different observations can then be expressed in a direct or indirect manner.

11.6.1. DIRECT CALCULATIONS OF OBSERVER VARIABILITY

In the direct form of expression, each pair of observations is compared individually in a calculation that forms an increment, ratio, or some other specific expression denoting their agreement (or disagreement). For example, if a particular person is rated as having 10.2 units by Observer A and 14.3 units by Observer B, the disagreement can be cited as an increment of 4.1 (= 14.3−10.2) units. Although the incremental technique is the most straightforward approach, several other mathematical methods can also be used. One appealing mechanism, intended to standardize the results, is to cite the incremental difference as a proportion of the average value. Thus, in the example just cited, the average value of the two observers is 12.25 (=[10.2+14.3]/2). The proportionate disagreement would be $4.1/12.25 = .335$. After these individual expressions are determined for each pair of observations, their average value for the entire group can be determined as a direct expression of observed consistency.

To avoid having positive and negative values cancel one another, the individual values are commonly analyzed, in a manner analogous to the calculation of standard deviations, by squaring the results, adding them, finding the average value of the sum, and then taking its square root. Thus, if d_i represents the value of the individual disagreement for the i-th pair in a set of data containing n pairs, the average disagreement would be $\sqrt{\Sigma d_i^2/n}$.

11.6.1.1. *Magnitudes of Individual Disagreement*

The process just described works quite well when the basic data are expressed in dimensional or quasi-dimensional values. For data expressed in ordinal grades, disagreements can be cited according to the number of categories of disparity. Thus, if one rating is **2+** and the other is **3+**, they differ by one grade; if one rating is **1+** and the other is **4+**, they differ by three grades. For binary data, where only two categories are available, four types of results can occur. For two observers, respectively, the two types of agreement are **YES-YES** and **NO-NO;** and the two types of disagreement are **YES-NO** and **NO-YES.**

11.6.1.2. *Disagreements in Nominal Data*

Although the values of nominal data cannot be ranked, ranks can sometimes be assigned to the disagreements in nominal categories. For example, the variable *birthplace in United States* contains 50 unrankable categories in a scale that cites 50 states. In a study of observer variability, however, a disagreement between **Maine** and **California** would be much greater than a disagreement between **Maine** and **New Hampshire.**

The magnitude of these nominal disagreements can be assigned arbitrary values, and the results can then be managed as though the arbitrary values represented quasi-dimensional data. This type of approach was used in a study of observer variability among histopathologists rating the cellular type of a series of lung cancers.[42] At one extreme, a minor disagreement between **well-differentiated adenocarcinoma** and **moderately well-differentiated adenocarcinoma** was rated as 0.5 units; at the other extreme, a major disagreement between **well-differentiated adenocarcinoma** and **well-differentiated epidermoid carcinoma** was rated as 2.5 units.

11.6.1.3. *Summary Expressions for Categorical Agreements*

For ordinal, binary, or nominal data, the most common summary expression of results is the *percentage agreement*. The number of exact agreements is divided by the total number of paired observations. Thus, if two observers completely agree on 37 of 50 paired observations, the percentage agreement is 74%.

This expression is satisfactory for binary data, but it does not reflect the magnitude of the categories of disagreement in ordinal or nominal data. For nominal data, this magnitude can be summarized, as noted in the preceding section, by assigning arbitrary values to the disagreements and finding their average magnitude. For ordinal data, the magnitude of discrepancy in categories can also be assigned arbitrary values, and the results can be cited as an expression of *weighted percentage agreement*. An example of this procedure is shown in Kramer and Feinstein's discussion of biostatistical indexes of concordance.[105]

11.6.2. INDIRECT COEFFICIENTS

In the indirect method of expression, the entire pattern of paired agreements and disagreements is cited with a statistical coefficient of association. The coefficient expresses the relationship between the observed results and the results expected from a particular mathematical model.

11.6.2.1. *Coefficients of Correlation*

The most familiar mathematical model used for dimensional data determines a correlation coefficient for the straight line that best fits the standardized data. A value near 1 for this coefficient indicates a close relationship between the two sets of observations; a value near 0 indicates little or no relationship. Correlation coefficients can also be calculated, using the observed results and the values expected under the null hypothesis of no relationship, for the associations found in categorical data.

11.6.2.2. *Coefficients of Concordance*

Although correlation coefficients have become standard statistical expressions of agreement, the coefficients indicate trends rather than concordance.[105] For example, if one procedure yields results that are always twice as high as the other, or always 10 units higher, the two sets of observations never achieve agreement, but they will have a perfect r value of 1.

In dimensional data, a close correlation will allow the value of one variable to be easily converted into the value of the other. Such correlations have been used by chemical laboratories as a standard procedure for mutual transformations in which a dimensional result measured by one method is converted to the result obtained by some other method. When the correlation is close enough, the conversion process is accurate and effective. (In circumstances where the investigator is specifically concerned with agreement rather than trend in dimensional data, the intraclass correlation coefficient can be substituted for the ordinary correlation coefficient.)[65]

For non-dimensional data, however, the correlation coefficient that expresses a trend among two sets of categorical observations does not allow their corresponding values to be mutually transformed and may not express their actual agreement. Consequently, agreement—particularly for non-dimensional data—is best expressed statistically with a coefficient of concordance, rather than trend. Coefficients of concordance are also desirable because they make provision for the proportions of agreement that might be expected to occur by chance alone from the patterns of ratings given by the compared observers.

For binary data, the best indirect coefficient of concordance is kappa, and for ordinal data, weighted kappa. No quantitative standards have been established for the level at which a concordance is considered good, excellent, etc. For kappa, however, Landis and Koch[109] have suggested the following guidelines:

Value of Kappa	*Strength of Agreement*
< 0	Poor
0–.20	Slight
.21–.40	Fair
.41–.60	Moderate
.61–.80	Substantial
.81–1.00	Almost perfect

The statistical methods of calculating these coefficients of concordance have been described and illustrated elsewhere.[65,105]

11.6.2.3. *"Head-to-Head" vs. "Side-to-Side" Analyses*

A statistical evaluation of concordance sometimes becomes ineffectual because the results are analyzed in a "side-by-side" rather than "head-to-head" manner. For example, suppose Observers A and B have each been asked to examine the retina of 100 patients and to rate each retina as being **normal** or **abnormal.** In one format of expression, the results could be cited as follows:

Observer	Observer A		Total
B	**Normal**	**Abnormal**	*Total*
Normal	45	28	73
Abnormal	7	20	27
Total	52	48	100

In a second format of expression, the results could be tabulated as:

	Normal	**Abnormal**	*Total*
Observer A	52	48	100
Observer B	73	27	100
Total	125	75	200

In the first format, the analysis is matched so that the results are shown in a head-to-head manner. We can see each observer's ratings in simultaneous relationship to the ratings of the other observer. We can also cite the results with expressions of concordance, such as a percentage agreement of 65% ($= [45+20]/100$), and a kappa coefficient of .29. In the second format, the results are unmatched and presented in a side-by-side manner. All we can say is that the diagnosis of **normal** was made by Observer A in 52% of the patients and by Observer B in 73%. We cannot go any further in discussing the actual agreement of the two observers.

The value of a matched or head-to-head analysis is sometimes overlooked when investigators report studies of observer variability with the unmatched or side-by-side results.

11.6.3. EXPRESSIONS FOR MULTIPLE OBSERVERS

All of the foregoing statistical citations of concordance depended on the idea that a pair of observations was being evaluated for each entity. If more than two observations exist for each entity, the statistical process becomes much more complex. In one approach, a generalized index of correlation or concordance can be calculated to express the results for all observations on all entities.[65] A simpler approach, yielding results that are easier to understand, is to calculate the statistical expressions for each of the possible pairs of observers, and then to take the overall average of the pairwise results. For example, if data are available for Observers A, B, and C, we could calculate the kappa values for A vs. B, A vs. C, and B vs. C. The overall index—if one is desired—would be the average of these three kappa values.

11.6.4. INTERPRETATION OF THE STATISTICAL EXPRESSIONS

Despite the major advantages of any quantitative citation, statistical expressions of observer variability must be evaluated with careful qualitative judgment. The following important points (and pitfalls) should be kept in mind during those judgments.

1. The statistical expression depends entirely on the input challenge given to the observers and on the conditions in which the observations were made. This paramount feature of the field trial, as discussed later in Section 11.7 and in Chapter 13, is often neglected when the results are appraised exclusively according to the statistical numbers.

2. The statistical expression offers a *descriptive* account of the variability. Like other descriptive statistical expressions, the values of average increment, kappa, and other coefficients may be accompanied by confidence intervals, P values, or other inferential expressions that denote the stochastic fragility or stability of the numbers. Thus, an impressively high r value may not be statistically significant because the sample size was too small; conversely, an r value that is unimpressive or so low as to suggest no relationship may become statistically significant because of a huge sample size. Regardless of what is cited in the stochastic accompaniment of P values and confidence intervals, the main item to be evaluated for describing observer variability is the descriptive statistic, not the stochastic adornments.[57,105]

3. None of the existing statistical methods of expression is ideal. The direct calculations provide a summary of the results, but they do not indicate the pattern of the relationship and they do not contain provision for agreements that might occur by chance alone. The indirect coefficients indicate the pattern of the relationship, but individual distinctions are lost. The coefficients of correlation show trends, rather than agreements, and contain no provision for the effects of chance agreement. The coefficients of concordance, which show the total pattern of agreement and which make provision for the role of chance agreement, can be affected by numerical features—analogous to prevalence of disease in diagnostic marker tests—of the group of entities used as the input challenge.[65,104]

For all these reasons, the statistical expressions offer an invaluable numerical summary of observer variability, but the number must be interpreted with thoughtful judgment about what it represents and what lies behind it.

11.7. Decisions About the Need for Field Trials of Observer Variability

As noted earlier, many clinimetric indexes have never received field trials of observer variability because the investigators developed the index, felt reassured by their appraisals of its sensibility and by the results noted in pilot studies, and then proceeded to use the index in specific acts of research that helped demonstrate the value and "validity" of the index. A subsequent evaluator of the index might then be horrified to find that its observer variability had never been tested.

This horror is sometimes fully justified, but it is often overemphasized. If an index seems to have excellent sensibility, if its substantial value is immediately apparent, and if its pilot studies and routine clinical application seem to indicate no major discrepancies in its use, the organization of a formal field trial of observer variability may be a supererogatory item of scientific window dressing. Although the trials might show certain inconsistencies among different users, the values for such coefficients as kappa would probably be above .6, thereby indicating a substantial agreement that was already recognized before the trial. The results might satisfy the quantitative desires of a rigorous evaluator, but a clinical investigator might believe that the trials were not a particularly productive way to use time, effort, and resources in clinical research.

Although this type of clinical judgment is sometimes warranted in decisions to avoid (or reject) a field trial of observer variability, the decisions are often unjustified; and field trials are often necessary or desirable in many circumstances where they have not been conducted. For example, whenever specific studies have been done of observer variability among histopathologists and diagnostic radiologists, the results have sometimes been comforting, but have often revealed shocking inconsistencies.[42]

A field trial of observer variability seems particularly necessary whenever the use of the index requires important judgmental rather than factual decisions. For example, suppose the index calls for someone to be designated as **old** if age is above 70 years. This decision can be carried out with minimal variability. If the designation of **old** is to be given to someone who "looks old," different observers may vary greatly in the way they carry out this decision for different people. Thus, in an excellent study of the problems, Hutchinson et al.[91] have recently shown that judgmental rather than factual decisions were the prime sources of variability in the use of an index intended to categorize the likelihood that a particular clinical event was an adverse drug reaction.

Because both the Apgar Score and the TNM staging system depend on a relatively straightforward classification of direct clinical observations, they involve relatively little judgment, and they can be used with relatively high consistency. On the other hand, new developments in diagnostic imaging may create major inconsistencies in the future use of TNM staging systems. Because the results of radionuclide or other scans are often interpreted by the radiologist as being **negative, equivocal,** or **positive** for evidence of tumor, and because the existing TNM criteria offer no guidance on how to classify the **equivocal** results, a particular patient's TNM stage will differ substantially according to whether the equivocal results are regarded as negative or positive by different clinical raters.[58]

The decision about when a field trial of observer variability is necessary will therefore depend on a close scrutiny of what the index contains and how it is constructed. If the ingredients of the index can easily receive different interpretations by different users, or if substantial judgmental decisions are involved in identifying or combining the ingredients, a field trial should be carried out to add quantitative reassurance to qualitative beliefs about sensibility. If a field trial has not been conducted, however, an evaluator should also think carefully about the need for such a trial before reflexively condemning an index that has not received one.

Chapter 12

The Evaluation of Validity

Validity is probably the most difficult word encountered in the -metrics of clinical and psychosocial indexes. The word commonly appears in ordinary language, but is given special meanings for its -metric usages, and the usages include a variety of things that are cited with different prefixes. Someone who has already developed ideas about *validity* from previous experience with the word may find that the ideas have been substantially altered in the professional jargon. When the jargon adds an array of prefixes to differentiate various types of validity—such as *face validity, content validity, criterion validity,* and *construct validity*—substantial effort may be needed simply to distinguish and remember all the different connotations.

Perhaps the greatest problem, however, is that the same word, *validity,* can be applied to characterize the three different goals of scientific measurement, which are usually labeled as *consistency, accuracy,* and *suitability.* The attempt to cover all three objectives with a single word creates the different varieties of validity, and evokes the plethora of confusing adjectives used to denote the distinctions.

12.1 Components of Validity

The ideas previously discussed for consistency, accuracy, and suitability appear in different ways as component parts of validity.

12.1.1. CONSISTENCY

The appraisal of consistency, as discussed in Chapter 11, is often regarded as a separate act of evaluation, different from what is done to

190

appraise validity. Nevertheless, when critics or potential users ask if an index has been validated, they usually want to know about consistency as well as the other aspects of validity. The basic idea behind the question is that an inconsistent index will not be valuable or useful, regardless of how well it scores in any other tests of validity.

Having been discussed in Chapter 11, and not being part of the customary evaluations of validity, consistency will not receive further attention here. It is mentioned now, however, to note that consistency (or reliability) is often regarded as a component of the "validation" process.

12.1.2. ACCURACY

The idea of accuracy is familiar and easy for most scientists. It is readily determined for laboratory measurements of chemical or other appropriate substances by noting the closeness with which the result of a particular procedure conforms to the result obtained with either a definitive standard or some other reference procedure that has measured the same entity. Despite its obvious virtues, however, *accuracy* is a major problem in clinical and psychosocial indexes, because of the many circumstances—noted in the next two sections—in which a definitive standard either does not exist or cannot be readily used.

12.1.2.1. *Absence of a Definitive Standard*

For certain types of clinical measurements, a definitive standard may not exist, or the index itself may become the definitive standard. For example, when a cytologist makes a diagnosis of cancer from a Pap smear, we can use the interpretation of the tissue biopsy as a definitive standard. On the other hand, when different histopathologists designate the cellular type of tissue for a particular cancer, we do not have a single definitive standard for the interpretation, unless one of the pathologists is accorded the deified status of unquestioned authority.

A definitive standard also does not exist for many indexes that are expressed in an ordinal scale of arbitrary grades. Thus, there are no definitive standards for such indexes as the Apgar Score, the TNM stages of cancer, the Glasgow Coma Scale, the New York Heart Association Functional Classification, the Katz Index of Activities of Daily Living, or any of the diverse clinical indexes that are cited in such global scales as **trace, mild, moderate, severe,** or **0, 1+, 2+, 3+, 4+.** In all of these examples, the rating given to the phenomenon is what we use because no definitive measurement exists.

In other circumstances, the index itself may create the definitive standard, thereby having nothing against which to be tested. For example, when a clinician uses diagnostic criteria to make a clinical diagnosis of coronary artery disease, we can check the accuracy of the diagnosis against the more definitive findings noted at coronary angiography, surgery, or necropsy. On the other hand, when appropriate diagnostic criteria are used as clinical indexes for making a diagnosis of rheumatic fever, rheumatoid arthritis, or systemic lupus erythematosus, the criteria themselves provide the definitive standard, and no external mechanism is available for checking the results. Some other clinicians may disagree with the contents of the criteria or with the results obtained in individual patients, but a definitive external standard is not available for confirmation or refutation.

12.1.2.2. *Conformity with Consensual Standards*

The absence of a definitive standard need not deter the assessment of accuracy if an investigator makes the necessary efforts and adjustments. The effort involves the development of a mechanism to create a reference standard, and the adjustment involves a willingness to recognize that what becomes tested is conformity rather than accuracy.

The most common mechanism used to create a reference standard is a process that is often called *consensual validation*. For this process, a group of appropriate authorities is assembled. They deliberate over the particular issue at hand and agree on what will be regarded as the correct or standard result. The process can be conducted in diverse ways, some of which have been given titles such as *Delphi technique* and *nominal group formation*.[64]

The consensual process can be used to establish standards for a wide array of indexes, ranging from a definitive diagnosis of a histopathologic tissue to a graded rating of a patient's clinical condition. This same process is constantly used, although not often recognized as such, when a committee establishes the "correct" answers for the questions asked in an examination certifying a clinician's competence, or when criteria are developed to rate performance in an audit of a clinician's quality of care.

After the standard is consensually established, we can check the degree of conformity it has received from the tested procedure (or performer). The performance can be graded for its correctness or "goodness," but the term *accuracy* is not really appropriate for the arbitrary standards. Besides, accuracy is usually regarded as a permanent trait, whereas correctness is subject to change according to the authorities who establish the standards. For example, the correct answer to a particular question in a specialty-board examination can vary from one era to the next; and a plan of clinical management that was rated as good in one year may be rated as poor several years later.

The idea of creating definitive standards by using a consensus of authorities may be viewed with disdain by scientists who are accustomed to testing hard data for accuracy. This type of consensus, however, was used—as discussed earlier in Section 11.1.2—to establish the basic dimensions of such fundamental hard data as the length of a meter, volume of a liter, weight of a gram, etc. Furthermore, a consensual type of process is also used routinely for establishing the definitive result in laboratory measurements. In most good laboratories, each measurement of a particular entity is usually repeated once or twice, and the correct result is taken to be the consensus of those measurements, often calculated as a mean for two values or as the mean of the closest two of three.

The differences found in a large number of individual measurements performed to reach such a consensus were, in fact, the source of what is now called a Gaussian (or "normal") curve of distribution for statistical data.[43] After noting the disagreements that occurred when the same measurement process was repeated for the same entity, Gauss decided that the "correct" value would be the consensus of the measurements—i.e., the mean. He then found that the "errors," i.e., the deviations from the mean, were distributed in the pattern that now bears his eponym.

The strategy of setting standards by consensus is thus well established for hard data and is readily applicable for the hardening of soft data. The main problem in the strategy is not the idea of using a consensus but the difficulty of getting a suitable group of authorities whose statements or opinions will form the consensus.

12.1.3. SUITABILITY

Problems of suitability seldom arise for the customary measurements performed in scientific laboratories. If we decide to measure serum molybdenum or urinary yttrium, we measure it "because it is there." If the measurement process is consistent and accurate, the laboratory has done its job well, and someone else can then worry about how to use the information.

Most clinical indexes, however, are constructed to serve a particular purpose, and an index cannot be regarded as satisfactory unless it actually serves that purpose. The suitability of the index in accomplishing its clinical purpose is therefore an important component of validity, although seldom needed in most appraisals of *quality control* or other evaluations for laboratory data. For example, suppose we have developed a highly consistent and accurate method of measuring body temperature or the size of the pupils of the eye. Despite impressive consistency and accuracy, neither measurement would be a suitable index of pain, anxiety, or functional capacity.

Many of the most important issues in judging suitability were discussed in Chapter 10 when we considered the sensibility of an index. The judgments were almost all qualitative, involving the application of enlightened common sense, with no statistical tactics. The attributes evaluated with this type of qualitative appraisal are usually called *face validity,* in reference to what is noted with a simple inspection of the basic idea of an index, and *content validity,* when the appraisal takes a deeper look into the component elements and structure of the index. Thus, by overt inspection we would reject the face validity of an index that uses pupil size alone to denote a person's functional capacity. If the index of functional capacity contains a composite of several components—a person's ability to work, the ability to perform daily activities without assistance, and the size of the pupils—the index seems basically aimed in the right direction, but its content validity is flawed by the inclusion of pupil size.

Suitability can also be evaluated, however, with quantitative methods. In these methods (which will be discussed in Section 12.3), statistical strategies are used to show that the constructed index is appropriate for its purpose. This appraisal is often called *construct validity.*

The two basic ideas that are examined in statistical tests of validity— accuracy and suitability—are discussed in greater detail in the two main sections that follow. The demonstration of accuracy in conforming to a reference standard is called *criterion validity* or *criterion-related validity* (Section 12.2). The demonstration that the index is suitable for its job is called *construct validity* (Section 12.3).

12.2. Criterion-Related Validity

Clinicians may sometimes have difficulty in deciding whether a particular type of validation represents *criterion validity* or *construct validity.* For example, suppose our laboratory measures the serum level of carcinoembryonic antigen (CEA) and we then use the result as a diagnostic marker for cancer of the colon. The CEA measurement can be checked for accuracy in two ways. In the first way, the result measured in our laboratory is compared with what is obtained when CEA in the same specimen is measured in a reference laboratory. In the second way, when the CEA result is used as a surrogate marker to denote the presence or absence of cancer of the colon, the accuracy of the marker is checked against the patient's definitive status, noted via other forms of examination, as having or not having cancer of the colon. Since both processes involve a determination of accuracy by comparison with a definitive standard, both processes might be regarded as tests of criterion validity.

In psychosocial use of the nomenclature, however, *criterion validity* usually refers to agreement with another measurement of exactly the same phenomenon. Thus, to test criterion validity, the measurement of CEA is compared in our laboratory and in the reference laboratory. *Construct validity,* in referring to the suitability of an index for its job, would be tested when we check the accuracy of CEA as a diagnostic marker. If the result of the index and the standard criterion measurement refer to the state of the examined entity at a single point in time, the relationship shows *concurrent validity.* If the criterion result is obtained at a future date, rather than concomitantly, the relationship to the index is called *predictive validity.*

As examples of the two types of timing, suppose we want to validate the score achieved by clinical candidates in a certifying examination given by a specialty board or medical licensing agency. If the reference standard consists of ratings given to the candidates just before the examination by the supervisors of the candidate's educational and training programs, we assess *concurrent validity.* If the reference standard consists of ratings given ten years later by patients, colleagues, or other evaluators, the results of the examination would be tested for *predictive validity.* In the architectural structures[54] used for the statistical studies, concurrent validity can easily be assessed from cross-sectional data. Predictive validity usually requires the more complex arrangements of longitudinal follow-up data in a cohort study.

12.2.1. STATISTICAL EXPRESSIONS

Most tests of criterion-related validity are cited with the same types of statistical expressions used in tests of consistency. When the scales of the clinimetric index and of the criterion variable are commensurate—i.e., having exactly the same categories of expression—the magnitudes of agreement (or disagreement) can be directly determined for each entity under observation. The results can then be cited in the direct forms of expression discussed in Section 11.6.1. The magnitudes of individual disagreement can be appropriately summarized or cited categorically in terms such as percentage agreement (or accuracy). With commensurate scales, the results can also be expressed indirectly with the coefficients of concordance[54,105] discussed in Section 11.6.2.2.

In many circumstances, however, the clinimetric index and the criterion variable may not be cited in commensurate scales. For example, a child's temperature might be estimated as **high fever, slight fever,** or **no fever** from a parent's palpation of the child's forehead. When the "palpation index" is checked against the child's dimensionally measured temperature, the two sets of results will have different scales. They can be assessed for concordance only if the temperature dimensions are arbitrarily demarcated into three ordinal zones that correspond to high, slight, or no fever. With noncommensurate scales, the only available statistical expression would be a correlation coefficient rather than a citation of concordance.

Other problems in the statistical assessment of accuracy arise when construct validity is tested for diagnostic markers, prognostic markers, and certain other clinical indexes. The problems—which involve management of uncertain results, choices of demarcation boundaries, and direct vs. indirect statistical expressions—will be discussed in Section 12.3.4.

12.2.2. COGNATE INDEXES AS SUBSTITUTES FOR CRITERION VARIABLES

When a definitive criterion is not available or has not been constructed by consensus, an existing "cognate" index—which measures the same or closely related phenomenon—is often used as a substitute criterion, particularly if the cognate index has achieved satisfactory acceptance and stature in its role. For example, suppose we have developed a new index that is faster or cheaper than other cognate indexes for rating a patient's functional capacity in activities of daily living. A definitive standard does not exist for this rating, but the other commonly used indexes (such as those developed by Katz[98] and by Barthel[120]) have become well accepted for this purpose. Accordingly, either one (or both) of these cognate indexes might be used as a substitute criterion variable for validating the new index.

When a new index shows close agreement with several cognate indexes that have been substituted as criterion variables, the total result is said to show *convergent validity*. This attribute is desirable if the new index is simpler or easier to use than the cognate indexes. Otherwise, a high value of convergent validity would raise questions about the utility of the new index. If it agrees so well with existing indexes, why is it needed? The latter question is commonly asked during the evaluation of construct validity, as discussed in Section 12.3.3.2, when we try to show that a new index has discriminating value (or "discriminant validity") by *not* having a high correlation with existing cognate indexes.

12.2.3. INFORMAL APPRAISALS OF CRITERION VALIDITY

The last point to be noted in this discussion of criterion-related validity is that it is often *not* formally tested for clinimetric indexes. In contrast to psychosocial indexes, many clinimetric indexes are constructed to provide a direct expression of an observed phenomenon that is either tangible or quasi-tangible. Because the index is intended to describe or designate that phenomenon, the correlation between the index and the phenomenon is usually developed while the index is being created, and further tests of the co-relationship may then seem unnecessary.

For example, no panels of authorities have ever been assembled to create consensual standards as reference criteria that might be used in correlations or other analyses intended to validate the Apgar score of a newborn baby's condition, the TNM Staging for spread of a cancer, or the New York Heart Association Criteria for a patient's functional capacity. Because these indexes were developed in direct association with the depicted phenomena, and because the indexes seem sensible and seem to work well in pilot studies or actual practice, they have not received tests of criterion-related validity.

The validation of these indexes has usually occurred not from checking them directly against a reference criterion but from the construct validity they achieved when applied in other forms of research.

12.3. Construct Validity

Construct validity has always been a difficult concept for clinicians to understand because the word *construct* is seldom used in clinical activities, and because the concept involves a quantitative attempt to evaluate something that clinicians usually assess either with qualitative judgment or with quantitative strategies that are not called *construct validity*.

12.3.1. THE CONCEPT OF A CONSTRUCT

Although *construct validity* is an unfamiliar term, clinicians frequently engage in the process of validating constructs. The process seems unfamiliar mainly because the clinician's constructs are not called *constructs*, and because the validation often occurs in a different location in the analytic sequence of -metric research.

The things that clinicians regard as a *disease*, as *normal*, as *decompensation* of an organ or system, as an *excess* or *deficiency* of a particular substance, or as *severity* of an illness are all *constructs*. These things do not exist as discrete overt entities of nature, like a tree or a chemical element. Instead, they are created intellectually as conceptual ideas, labels, or explanations for observed phenomena.

A new construct is established or developed when clinicians decide to alter the concept of a disease, such as the changes that eliminated the nineteenth-century diagnoses of *consumption, dropsy,* and *chlorosis;* when new diseases are identified, such as Acquired Immune Deficiency Syndrome, Toxic Shock Syndrome, or Lyme Disease; or when new pathophysiologic mechanisms are discovered, such as the roles of DNA, T-cell and B-cell lymphocytes, and pre-load and after-load cardiovascular dynamics in human biology.

In all these and many other circumstances, clinicians develop and incorporate new constructs into clinical reasoning. Because of the diverse microbiologic, biochemical, physiologic, pathologic, epidemiologic, and other activities that occur in medical science, all of these constructs become established and their existence becomes validated by research that is done before (or while) the construct enters the day-to-day work of clinical medicine. By the time clinimetric efforts are instituted to develop an index for identifying the construct diagnostically, for grading its magnitude, or for indicating changes in its state from one occasion to another, the construct itself has already become well accepted, and clinicians are accustomed to thinking about it.

12.3.2. CONCEPTS OF CONSTRUCT VALIDITY

The idea of *construct validity* originally referred to an appraisal of the effectiveness with which an index did its job in describing an existing or established construct. The idea was later expanded, however, to include two additional challenges. One of these challenges occurs when a construct does not previously exist and is newly created by an index. For example, among the many things people might say when talking about the weather many years ago, a wind-chill factor was seldom discussed until this idea was created by a formal index in meteorology. Once the idea was introduced, the wind-chill factor was promptly recognized and accepted as a useful, reasonable construct. In many other situations, however, a newly created construct may not always be immediately accepted. In such circumstances, construct validity can refer to a demonstration that the proposed construct actually exists. A different challenge in construct validity arises if a new index is supposed to contain or do something that makes it different from (and presumably better than) the existing cognate indexes. For this goal, construct validity can refer to the evidence showing that the new index is differentiated from the others.

These three concepts of construct validity—for appraising description, existence, or differentiation—are discussed further in the next three subsections.

12.3.2.1. *Descriptive Issues in Construct Validity*

If a construct such as congestive heart failure has already become established, an index that describes the idea should be relatively easy to appraise for *construct validity*. Having already developed their own informal expressions or judgments for describing the construct, clinicians can evaluate the sensibility of the clinimetric index by noting how well its formal structure corresponds to those informal expressions and judgments.

The evaluation process is relatively easy if universal agreement has already occurred about the ideas contained in the construct. Things may be more difficult if the construct itself is viewed in diverse ways by diverse people. For example, if we turn from ideas about disease and pathophysiology to issues in teaching and delivering clinical care, considerable disagreement may occur among different clinicians and patients about what is to be regarded as excellence in such constructs as *medical education, clinical competence, functional capacity,* or *quality of life.* In these situations, everyone usually agrees that the construct itself actually exists. The disagreements arise about what is to be included in the construct or demarcated as **excellent, good, fair, or poor.**

This problem in the contents of a well-accepted construct also occurs in psychosocial indexes. Everyone may agree about the existence of constructs such as *intelligence, racial prejudice,* and *familial interrelationships,* but major disagreements may occur about the way in which the construct is identified and demarcated in an index. For example, the methods of measuring intelligence have been an ongoing source of unresolved dispute among psychosocial scientists.[70] The psychosocial arguments—which usually rest on judgments about suitability of the selected components, aggregations, and scales—can sometimes be resolved with the principles of sensibility discussed in Chapter 10.

12.3.2.2. *Validation of Post-Analytic Constructs*

In clinical work, most constructs are established before an index is developed to describe them, and relatively few constructs have been created, like the wind-chill factor, directly from the analysis of a newly formulated index. (An exception is the "double product index" of cardiac status, obtained when pulse rate and systolic blood pressure are multiplied.)

Post-analytic constructs are particularly likely to arise if a mathematical model—such as factor analysis or some other multivariate process—is used to choose certain cogent aggregates that become designated as *factors, principal components,* or *clusters.* These cogent aggregates, which are identified in retrospect after the data were analyzed, may then be regarded and labeled as *constructs.* Thus, a psychosocial investigator may decide that a certain set of aggregated ingredients represents a *maternal-child-anxiety-interaction factor.* Analogously, from an analysis of results in a multiple-choice examination for certification by a medical specialty board, the investigators may cull out an *elitist-education-scientific-humanism factor.*

In such circumstances, when the construct is developed after rather than before the index is created, the investigator may have difficulty persuading people that the new, arbitrarily produced construct is correct, useful, and valuable. A demonstration of *construct validity* may then be needed to convince other people that there actually exists an entity such as a *maternal-child-anxiety-interaction factor* or an *elitist-education-scientific-humanism factor.*

12.3.2.3.   *Differential Attributes of a Construct*

Suppose severity of illness for a particular disease is described according to the magnitude of symptoms produced by that disease only. A patient in whom the disease is discovered during a screening test, and who is extremely sick or even moribund because of the concomitant effects of co-morbid ailments, might nevertheless be described by the index as **asymptomatic.** To avoid this type of incongruity, a patient's severity of illness would not be regarded as well described if the index depends only on the status of a single disease. A suitable new index for the construct of severity of illness would have to include components referring to co-morbidity, as well as components for the main disease under consideration.

If the old index of severity of illness had its contents expanded to include an additional rating for severity of co-morbidity, we would immediately recognize that the new index is superior to the old one for describing the condition of patients rather than the state of a main disease alone. On the other hand, when the two indexes are used in a large group of patients with the main disease, the two indexes will often yield similar results for the many patients who have only the single main disease, without any significant co-morbidity. Consequently, the two indexes would often agree with each other and would have a reasonably high degree of statistical correlation. The instances in which the two results disagree in patients with major co-morbidity, however, would be particularly valuable for showing the effectiveness of the new index. The disagreements would be the main evidence that the new index discerns something that is undetected with the old index.

Therefore, when a new index is intended to be reasonably similar to an old one, but to do something distinctively different, the statistical correlation of construct validity plays an interesting double role. To show that the two indexes are reasonably similar, we would want a suitably high degree of association, but to show that the two indexes are different, we do not want the association to be too high. The *dissociation* is the feature that will demonstrate the desired difference. The measurement of dissociation is further discussed in Section 12.3.4.2.

12.3.2.4. *Clinical Approaches to Construct Validity*

Almost all the indexes used in clinical practice were developed in the conventional pre-analytic manner rather than with a retrospective post-analytic technique. Because the construct had already become well accepted, there was no need to prove the existence of the construct itself; and the quality of description in the index was readily appraised with principles of sensibility, using qualitative clinical judgment. If a new index was formulated to include things that were missing or inadequately managed in an old index, the distinctive contributions of the new index would also be appraised with sensible judgment.

For all these reasons, most clinicians have seldom encountered a formal evaluation of *construct validity,* and may never have heard of the idea until it is introduced to them by a psychosocial consultant. The introduction may occur when the consultant is invited to collaborate in developing a new clinical index, such as a measurement of satisfaction with medical care, or when the clinician is first confronted by the statistical procedures used for "psychometric" analysis of the results of medical licensure or specialty-board examinations. Unfamiliar with the concept and confused by the statistical expressions, the clinician may abandon (or fail to use) the qualitative judgment needed for important decisions about construct validity. These decisions include answers to questions such as when (or whether) construct validity should be checked and what methods should be used to check it.

12.3.3. CONSTRUCT VALIDITY AS A SUBSTITUTE FOR CRITERION-RELATED VALIDITY

Although the appraisal of validity is particularly important if a construct was generated rather than described by the data used to develop an index, the evaluation of construct validity has another major role in -metric strategy. If criterion validity cannot be tested because a reference criterion is not available (or not used), construct validity is often substituted as the main focus of quantitative statistical appraisals.

This type of substitution can occur in several types of circumstances where a reference criterion is not employed. The circumstances include situations in which a reference criterion is impossible or unfeasible to create; or when the reference criterion is co-opted by the index itself, achievable but not developed, developed but not readily available, or developed and available but disregarded. These different no-criterion situations are briefly outlined in the next few subsections.

12.3.3.1. *Reference Criterion Impossible*

When a patient describes the existence of a symptom such as chest pain, abdominal pain, menstrual cramps, or trouble in urinating, a direct reference criterion may be impossible to establish. We can do various things to decide whether the patient is a reliable reporter; we can try various "tricks" in questioning or testing the symptom; and we can observe various associated phenomena that may help support or deny the patient's statement—but no external criterion is available to confirm the statement directly. We can accept it or reject it, but it cannot be validated with an external criterion.

12.3.3.2. *Reference Criterion Unfeasible*

Although many reference criteria can be created with the consensual process described in Section 12.1.2.2, the process may be so difficult to carry out that it becomes unfeasible. For example, a group of authorities may have little difficulty reaching agreement about standards for diagnosing myocardial infarction or for grading severity of congestive heart failure, but consensus may be difficult (and sometimes impossible) to achieve for standards of medical education, quality of life, satisfaction with health care, or maternal-child anxiety interactions.

12.3.3.3. *Reference Criterion Co-opted*

For certain types of diagnostic criteria or for other situations in which the clinimetric index becomes the reference standard, no external criterion can be tested. The index has taken on or co-opted the role as criterion variable.

This situation was illustrated in Section 12.1.2.1, with the indexes used as criteria for diagnosis of rheumatoid arthritis, systemic lupus erythematosus, and acute rheumatic fever. Other examples include the criteria used to diagnose diabetes mellitus from a glucose tolerance test, and all of the criteria that offer specifications for the diagnosis of psychiatric ailments, for the many maladies designated as syndromes rather than diseases, and for any other diagnoses of conditions that cannot be identified with objective pathognomonic evidence. If the designation of a disease requires a mixture of clinical and paraclinical information, the diagnostic criteria will also take the role of reference standard.

12.3.3.4. *Reference Criterion Achievable but Not Developed*

In this situation, as discussed earlier, reference criteria would be relatively easy to achieve, but suitable efforts have not yet been made. The absence of such efforts may be due merely to scientific oversight or neglect. More commonly, however, the investigators may be persuaded by other evidence of the index's validity and may believe that special efforts to quantify the validity are not worthwhile.

This situation commonly arises when the clinimetric index produces an adjective, describing the relative magnitude or grade of an entity, rather than a noun, indicating the existence of the entity. Thus, the diagnostic criteria cited in Section 12.3.3.3 create nouns that show the presence or absence of a particular disease, whereas the Apgar Score, TNM stages, New York Heart Functional Classification, and Glasgow Coma Scale all produce adjectives for the graded magnitude of a particular condition. Adjectives are produced by most psychosocial indexes—such as those concerned with attitudes, anxiety, depression, and family-support systems—and also by the many clinical ratings of magnitude for pain, dyspnea, menstrual cramps, dyschezia, and other subjective symptoms.

These clinical indexes of gradation are often established, after considerable thought and deliberation, by an individual expert or group of authorities. The person(s) who created the index may then believe that the deliberations and consensus about what went into the index have already provided enough validation, and that a separate panel of authorities need not be assembled for the additional formal activity of developing an independent consensus and testing the index against the consensual criteria. Instead, the developer(s) of the index may turn immediately to the direct applications or other forms of research, discussed later in Section 12.4, that help demonstrate the actual value, if not the formal criterion validity, of the index.

12.3.3.5. *Reference Criterion Developed but Not Readily Available*

Suppose we want to determine the accuracy of sputum Pap smears as indexes of the presence and histologic type of lung cancer. For a thorough test of criterion validity, we would need suitable biopsies of lung tissue for each patient entered in the study. Since the biopsies might not be attainable for all patients and might be deemed unnecessary or unethical for patients with negative roentgenograms and Pap smears, the result of the reference criterion will not always be known. If we eliminate the patients for whom a reference value is unavailable, the study may be marred by the problems of "work-up bias."[54] Accordingly, if we still want to test the criterion validity of the sputum

Pap smear, something other than histologic tissue will have to be used as a substitute criterion. For example, we might establish the concurrent absence of lung cancer by consensual validation, or by following the patient's clinical course to demonstrate that lung cancer did not develop.

A similar type of problem occurs when we want to achieve criterion validity for the results of a diagnostic index such as the results of computerized tomography or magnetic resonance imaging. The surgery or necropsy needed to show the true state of the tissue may not have been done in each patient. Consequently, because data from a standard criterion may not always be available, something else will have to be used instead if we want a routine appraisal of criterion validity.

12.3.3.6. *Reference Criterion Available but Disregarded*

In the last situation to be cited, a reference criterion is developed and available, but is disregarded. Sometimes the criterion is disdained because it depends on soft or possibly biased data, such as a program director's rating of clinical competence for a candidate taking a medical board certification examination. More commonly, however, the criterion is disregarded because it seems inappropriate for the purpose of the index or because the investigator is eager to begin using the index in further research rather than conducting "sterile" studies of criterion validity.

For example, a clinical index of a patient's functional capacity might be validated against the patient's performance in an exercise stress test, but the investigator might decide that the laboratory conditions of the stress test are not appropriate for establishing the patient's capacity in meeting the diverse challenges of everyday life. Alternatively, if functional capacity is to be used as an index of prognosis or change in a study of therapy, the investigator may want to proceed directly to the therapeutic research without pausing for the delay needed to conduct further clinimetric testing. This type of "validation by application," as discussed in Section 12.3.4.1, may often replace criterion validity but can also be tested in addition.

12.3.4. STRATEGIES OF CONSTRUCT VALIDATION

Construct validity can be appraised with at least two strategies. The first strategy—validation by application—is readily familiar to clinical scientists. It consists of seeing what happens when the index is used for its intended purpose in identifying, discriminating, predicting, or instructing. The second strategy, which might be called "distinctive dissociations," is used to show that the index does things that are distinctively different from what is done by existing cognate indexes.

An additional strategy, which provides evidence sometimes used to support the idea of construct validity, was discussed earlier in Section 11.5.2, as part of the evaluation of internal consistency. The strategy demonstrates the homogeneous coherence of the component parts of the index.

12.3.4.1. *Validation by Application*

Perhaps the most common type of validation for clinimetric indexes is constantly carried out by clinicians who do not know that the process constitutes an appraisal of *construct validity*. This type of appraisal occurs when the index is checked in the actual performance of its assigned job. For example, an index for rating status or changes in pain receives construct validation when it shows substantial differences that cogently distinguish the effects of the active and placebo treatments used in a clinical trial of analgesia. An index for rating clinical severity of illness may have its construct validity demonstrated predictively if its categories show a distinct prognostic gradient in patients' survival. The construct validity might be demonstrated concurrently if the index of severity shows that groups of cancer patients first treated with chemotherapy are substantially sicker than those chosen to receive radiotherapy. To demonstrate the construct validity of the Apgar Score, an investigator might use it to confirm the research hypothesis that the babies born at Hospital A are often in worse (or better) condition than the babies born at Hospital B.

An example of the clinical importance of validation by application was recently shown for a new clinical index for rating the severity of dyspnea.[118] Although the new index had been shown to have both criterion validity (in comparison with standard measurements of pulmonary function) and differential construct validity (in demonstrating things that could not be measured with pulmonary function tests), the index was initially given an apathetic reception by pulmonary specialists. Later on, however, the index became enthusiastically welcomed when a different aspect of its construct validity was shown in a randomized trial of theophylline vs. placebo therapy for patients with chronic obstructive lung disease.[119] The results in favor of the active agent were statistically significant when measured with the new clinical index, but not with conventional laboratory tests of pulmonary function.

12.3.4.2. *Distinctive Dissociations*

When a suitable cognate index is used as a substitute for a criterion variable, the comparison may be intended to show that the results of the new index are in the same general neighborhood as the results of the existing cognate index. The magnitude of agreement desired between the cognate index and the new index will vary, however, with the purpose of the new index. If the new index is being proposed because it is cheaper or easier to use than a cognate index, while offering essentially the same information, a high level of agreement might be desired to show that the new index can readily replace the old one. On the other hand, if the new index contains different information or is intended for a different purpose, the index would not be expected to have an extremely high correlation with cognate indexes. If the correlation is too high, as noted in Section 12.3.2.3, the new index may not be doing anything new.

For example, to show that hematocrit is a useful new construct in measuring hematologic status, we might demonstrate that hematocrit correlates closely with the cognate measurements of hemoglobin and red blood count. If the correlation is too high, however, we might conclude that a measurement of hematocrit is redundant unless it is shown to have some other special functions. The results of hematocrit and the other two indexes should correlate well enough to show that the indexes are reasonably related to one another, but a certain amount of distinctive dissociation is desirable to demonstrate that hematocrit is measuring some different attributes. Analogously, we would expect to find a reasonable correlation between old indexes that measure the anatomic spread of a cancer and new indexes that measure the clinical severity of the associated symptoms. Unless the two sets of indexes have some distinctive dissociation, however, the severity of symptoms may not require a separate measurement.

This type of dissociation can readily be demonstrated if a specific variable is available to check the accuracy of the index in diagnostic or prognostic prediction. Thus, if anatomic and symptom-severity indexes are being used as predictors of prognosis in patients with cancer, they can be checked simultaneously for their statistical impact on survival rates. If a separate predictive outcome variable is not available, however, distinctiveness can be shown only by direct comparisons of values for the new index and old indexes.

Such a demonstration was recently provided for a new clinical index of severity of dyspnea.[118] Its single-state values were shown to correlate reasonably well with the paraclinical data of pulmonary function tests and particularly well with a measurement of 12-minute walking distance. The transition values of the dyspnea index, however, did not correlate well with changes in pulmonary function tests, and showed only a fair correlation with changes in 12-minute walking distance. The investigators offered the dissociations as evidence that the new index identified clinical phenomena that were not discerned with the cognate paraclinical indexes.

Although dissociations can offer important evidence of useful distinctions, two indexes may sometimes be dissociated because the new one is unsatisfactory rather than distinctive or superior. For example, suppose we decided to assess the clinical competence of medical house staff by using a written test of each candidate's knowledge of sporting events and motion picture stars. If the results of a field trial show a poor correlation between the sports-movie index and cognate ratings of competence provided by the candidate's clinical supervisors, a proponent of the new index might contend that it is valuable because it has measured something novel and different, rather than something irrelevant.

12.3.4.3. *Surrogate, Predictive, and Challenge-Set Validity*

The accuracy with which a diagnostic marker identifies a particular disease can be directly tested if the marker is used individually as a surrogate index but not if it is a component of a larger composite index. For example, the carcinoembryonic antigen (CEA) laboratory test was originally offered as a surrogate marker for cancer of the colon. The marker was then evaluated for the accuracy with which its positive and negative results identified patients who had other evidence for the definitive presence or absence of colonic cancer. With various enzymes used as diagnostic markers for myocardial infarction, however, the results do not have a surrogate role. The clinical diagnosis depends on a composite combination of laboratory, clinical, and electrocardiographic evidence. The laboratory tests can be evaluated for their individual or surrogate accuracy in making the diagnosis,[139] but the evaluations would not reflect the combinatorial way in which the tests are used in clinical practice. (Furthermore, the evaluation process would be biased if the results of the laboratory markers were incorporated into the data used for making the definitive diagnosis of myocardial infarction.)[54,135]

Even if a diagnostic marker has been suitably evaluated for its validity as a surrogate test some residual questions will remain about the general accuracy of the test. The usual source of this problem is that the diagnostic marker may have been initially examined and evaluated in a special group of patients whose data were conveniently available to the investigator. That special group of patients, however, may not necessarily represent the groups to whom the diagnostic marker test will later be applied. Many evaluators, therefore, will delay conclusions about the general validity of a diagnostic marker test until it has been further examined in a new group of patients, different from the group in whom the test was originally developed and checked.

This same type of problem arises with prognostic indexes. The index may have been originally developed, using clinical and/or statistical methods of multivariate analysis, from data for a particular group of patients who are sometimes called the *generating* or *development* set. The data analyzed during the generating process may also show prognostic gradients, reductions in variance, or other statistical evidence of the index's validity as a prognostic predictor. Nevertheless, many evaluators will not regard the index as having been fully validated until it shows similar prognostic gradients or reductions in variance in a new *challenge-set* group of patients, different from the group used as the generating set.

This type of *challenge-set validity* or *group-replication validity* is distinctly different from the ideas contained in most discussions of criterion validity or construct validity. The latter discussions are concerned with the types of data that are to be related and evaluated for decisions about "validity." In challenge-set validity, the emphasis is on the groups of patients contained in the evaluations. The subject will be further discussed in Chapter 13, when we consider the types of patients chosen for field trials of an index.

12.3.5. STATISTICAL EXPRESSIONS AND POLICIES

When construct validity is assessed for its correlation or dissociation, the results can be cited with conventional statistical expressions. In certain circumstances, however, construct validity involves a test of the index's accuracy in making a concurrent diagnosis or a prognostic prediction. Special statistical approaches may then be needed to express the index's accuracy or other accomplishments and to avoid distortions in the groups under analysis. For example, such terms as *sensitivity, specificity,* and *likelihood ratios* are commonly used to denote the accuracy of a diagnostic marker test in agreeing with the definitive diagnosis of the selected disease.[54] Indexes that produce a prognostic prediction can be checked for accuracy in individual patients and for the prognostic gradient noted among an ordinal array of categories, such as Stages I, II, III, and IV.

Beyond these issues in the choice of a statistical expression, several important decisions are needed to establish policies for choosing the data and patients to be included in the information subjected to statistical analysis. These policies require decisions about the management of uncertain results, the choice of demarcation boundaries, and the use of direct vs. indirect statistical expressions. Since the policies represent arbitrary judgments, and since none of them is universally accepted as established, they will merely be outlined here. More extensive accounts of the policies can be found elsewhere.[54,105]

12.3.5.1. *Management of Uncertain Results*

The first statistical policy requires a decision about what to do when the result of the clinimetric index is uncertain. For example, if a diagnostic marker test yields a result that is **equivocal,** should the patient be excluded or included in an evaluation of the marker's sensitivity and specificity? If the patient is included, what rating of agreement or disagreement should be given to the equivocal result? If patients with equivocal results are excluded—a common practice in contemporary research for diagnostic marker tests—the statistical calculations can be grossly misleading for the accuracy of the test.[54,135] If the equivocal group is included, however, the customary calculations of sensitivity and specificity may be impossible, and some other forms of statistical expression will be necessary.[54]

An analogous problem arises when the result of the definitive standard is uncertain. For example, the exercise stress test is often evaluated today as a diagnostic marker for coronary disease that is definitively diagnosed with coronary arteriography. If patients who have equivocal arteriograms (or who have not had arteriography) are excluded from the study in which the diagnostic marker is evaluated, the statistical calculations may be grossly misleading.

A different problem arises in studies of predictive validity when the patient's status is unknown or uncertain for the outcome event that is the definitive standard. The attempts to deal with this problem statistically in cohort research have led to several forms of "life-table" or "actuarial" analysis, to the need for deciding which type of analysis to use, and to the realization that different choices may produce substantial differences in the statistical appraisals.[54]

12.3.5.2. *Choices of Demarcations*

Clinicians usually think in categories when deciding that a patient is sick or well, very sick or slightly sick, hypertensive or not hypertensive, in need of treatment or not in need of treatment, needing Treatment A or Treatment B, improved or not improved after treatment. To arrive at these categorical decisions, clinicians will regularly seek information that is available in categorical form, and will often convert non-categorical data into categorical demarcations.

For example, suppose a clinical trial has been done to compare Treatment A vs. placebo in the treatment of hypertension. The results can be reported in at least two distinctly different ways. In the first way, we analyze the data in their original form. The results might show that the mean reduction in blood pressure was 10.7 mmHg with Treatment A and 2.1 mmHg with placebo, and that the difference is statistically significant. In the second way, we first delineate a standard for "success" in reduction of blood pressure; we then categorize each patient's achievement (or non-achievement) of the success; and we then might note that success was attained (with statistical significance) in 23% of patients who received Treatment A and in 6% of those who received placebo.

Either set of analyses is an acceptable way of presenting the results of the trial; both sets show that Treatment A is an efficacious agent; and both sets will be considered when a clinician makes decisions about treatment for a particular patient. Nevertheless, most clinicians—if forced to choose between the two sets of information—would prefer the categorical results cited in the second set of data. The categorical expressions would provide a predictive indication of what can be expected as the chance of success for individual patients, whereas the mean values allow no individual estimates.

Because judgment is involved in demarcating the boundaries and contents of categories such as success, many data analysts prefer to use the first type of statistical process. It allows the mean values for the two treatments to be calculated and compared without any judgmental decisions about demarcating success. In contrast, the second type of analysis requires a major demarcational judgment before any statistical calculations can begin. Despite this apparent disadvantage, the second type of analysis is more useful for clinical decisions. Because the formation of categories is a fundamental activity both for clinical reasoning and for the clinimetric indexes used in the reasoning, clinical analyses of data will often depend on categorical demarcations.

The way these demarcations are chosen can greatly affect the quantitative results obtained in assessments of criterion validity. For example, suppose we want to test the predictive accuracy of a staging system that acts as a prognostic index in patients with lung cancer, and suppose we demarcate survival at five years as the outcome event to be predicted. Because the overall five-year survival rate in patients with lung cancer is only 7%, we could achieve 93% accuracy by immediately predicting that everyone will be dead even if the staging system itself adds nothing to the prognostic estimations. To give the prognostic index a more suitable challenge, we would need to demarcate a different time point for the outcome event. Since the six-month survival rate in lung cancer is about 50%, the statistical appraisal of the index would be more effective if it is tested for predictions of six-month rather than five-year survival.

The choice of demarcation points for either the clinimetric index or the criterion variable (or both) is a crucial feature of scientific judgment in clinical assessments of criterion validity. A prominent example of the problems and challenges is shown by the elaborate mathematical strategies that have been developed to use receiver-operating-curve characteristics and likelihood ratios in the statistical evaluation of demarcations for diagnostic marker tests.[54]

12.3.5.3. *Direct vs. Indirect Expressions*

Regardless of what strategies are chosen to deal with uncertain data or to create demarcations of data, the statistical results can ultimately be expressed—as discussed in Chapter 8 and in Sections 11.6.1 and 11.6.2—with direct citations of what happened or with indirect coefficients of the relationship. The direct citations are usually preferable scientifically because they allow the actual evidence to be presented and inspected. They are not preferred statistically, however, because they often require arbitrary judgments about the categories in which the direct evidence is to be enumerated and tabulated.

The indirect statistical coefficients have the advantage of not requiring any categorical judgments, but the disadvantage of not displaying evidence of what happens. Thus, when seeing values for such coefficients as r, ϕ, R^2, or kappa, or when receiving numerical statements of proportionate reduction (or explanation) in variance, the clinician is given an indirect account of what occurred and may get a reasonably good idea of the relationship between the clinimetric index and the validating variables—but no direct evidence is presented for the actual quantitative accomplishments of the clinimetric index or for the particular clinical subgroups in whom the accomplishments occurred.

12.4. The Scientific Role of Field Trials

Almost everything discussed in the preceding sections depended on an analysis of data obtained in a field trial. The analyses may have involved simple qualitative judgments or elaborate mathematical calculations—but all of the decisions relied on the data produced by the trial.

Although the results of the quantitative calculations often receive prominent emphasis for evaluating the criterion or construct validity of an index, a more fundamental issue in basic scientific thought is the structure of the field trial itself. Was it planned and conducted in a way that warrants all the mathematical attention given to the data? The answer to this question is a crucial scientific issue in any type of -metric activity, but the question is often overlooked when statistical coefficients of validity (and reliability) become the center of investigative attention. The next chapter is concerned with the diverse issues that must be considered before the results of a field trial can be accepted as having enough scientific credibility to justify subsequent statistical conclusions.

Chapter 13

Design and Evaluation of Field Trials

Like any other form of research, a field trial of an index has a distinctive purpose and structure. The statistical results of the trial will be used to quantify the consistency or validity of the index, but the mathematical expressions are merely end-stage numbers. Like the numerical ratings that emerge from an index itself, the statistical ratings produced by a field trial must be appraised for many qualitative issues that lie behind the numbers and that determine their sensibility and acceptability.

This type of qualitative appraisal is often neglected when the numerical results of field trials are regarded as validation for an index. Satisfied by the statistical coefficients, the investigators (and subsequent reviewers) may give little or no attention to the many important non-quantitative distinctions that affect a trial's scientific credibility and pertinence.

Some of these distinctions can be evaluated before a trial is planned; others involve critical decisions about the trial's objectives; some arise from the structure of the trial; and yet others affect the appropriate interpretation of the results. The rest of this chapter is concerned with these distinctions in pre-trial evaluations, and in the objectives, structure, and interpretations of the trial itself.

13.1. Pre-Trial Evaluations

Many field trials have been inefficient or inadequate because they were conducted prematurely. The investigators proceeded to do the trial before they had suitably checked certain important attributes that can be determined beforehand while the index is being developed. If sensibility had been given adequate attention or if suitable pilot studies had preceded the field trial, many overt defects could have been detected and eliminated (or repaired) before the trial began.

13.1.1. REVIEW OF SENSIBILITY

All of the issues of sensibility discussed in Chapter 10 should be reviewed before a field trial is planned. The review can reveal problems that need attention; and even when no problems are apparent, the review can help identify the objectives to be sought in the trial.

Because most of the main issues to be considered in a review of sensibility were cited in Chapter 10, they will not be repeated here. A valuable new concept was recently added by Kasl[97] in discussing indexes that serve as "research prostheses" for classifying psychosocial events as "maneuvers" in public health research. Kasl pointed out that indexes describing the proficiency of a maneuver should have a suitable scope of components, but the components should not include effects of the maneuver itself. For example, an index that measures the magnitude of stressful life events should cover the full spectrum of potentially stressful events but should not include reactions that can occur as a later outcome of the stress. Thus, if alcoholism occurs as a consequence of stress, alcohol intake should not be included among the phenomena used to describe stress. Analogously, an index that measures the magnitude of exposure to tobacco smoke should include cigars and pipes as well as cigarettes and should differentiate between inhaling and not inhaling, but should omit components that refer to coughing or a sense of relaxation.

13.1.2. REVIEW OF CONSISTENCY AND VALIDITY

Since consistency and validity are prominent objectives to be appraised in a field trial, the preceding developmental studies can be checked to see how well they have prepared the index for this appraisal. For example, many problems in consistency can be avoided with a careful check of the instructions that provide replicability in usage of the index. The preceding pilot studies can also be reviewed for any defects in the instructions. If unclear or poorly understood, the instructions can be improved and retested in new pilot studies before the field trial is begun.

In validity, many problems can be avoided if the investigators check in advance to be sure that the people to be investigated in the field trial are the same kinds of people who were studied when the index was being developed. If the two sets of investigated groups seem highly disparate, a pilot study of the index in the new group might demonstrate major problems, which can be identified and solved before the field trial is conducted.

13.2. **Objectives of the Trial**

Because a field trial can be done to test the different types of consistency and validity discussed in Chapters 11 and 12, the particular objectives of the trial should be clearly defined beforehand. Unless the goals are well delineated, the trial may have an unsuitable design and may fail to achieve its purpose. This problem becomes particularly important if a single trial is aimed at too many targets or if the targets are not adequately specified.

13.2.1. STUDIES OF CONSISTENCY

In the customary clinimetric situation, a field trial of consistency is intended to discern observer variability in use of the index. Each member of the input group (patients, specimens, films, etc.) is submitted to each of the observers, and the results are analyzed for agreement.

To be scientifically satisfactory, the study must be suitable in the composition of the input group, in the choice of participating observers, and in the mechanism with which the observers do their job. In addition to basic suitability, each of the component parts of the study must be compared in conditions that are appropriately similar. For example, the entities under observation should be unchanged from one observer to the next; the setting in which the observations occur should be essentially the same for each set of observations; and the process should be conducted with blinding or other appropriate tactics to ensure that each observation is unaffected by previous results.

These fundamental attributes of the research architecture of a field trial have been discussed in detail elsewhere,[54] and will be further considered in Section 13.3.4. The main point to be noted now is simply that a high value of the statistical coefficient of agreement does not necessarily mean that the procedure is consistent, nor does a low value prove inconsistency. Unless the field trial was done with a satisfactory research plan, the statistical results will have no more credibility than other measurements obtained with inadequate methods.

The problems of planning and executing a suitably designed field trial may be another reason so many clinimetric indexes have not been tested for observer variability. After noting the poor scientific quality of many existing field trials, and after meditating about all the things that must be done to create a good one, an investigator may decide to omit a formal test of observer variability and to go directly to studies of validity. These decisions are usually made with the hope that the existing judgmental appraisals and pilot studies will suffice to give the index a satisfactory degree of consistency. This hope is sometimes justified and even confirmed; but in other circumstances, a properly conducted field trial may demonstrate a disappointingly low consistency in use of the index.

Another problem that often militates against field trials of consistency is the frequent difficulty (or impossibility) of carrying out a good study of observer variability. The field trial is easy to do if the entities under observation are tangible, preservable, and readily sent for examination at whatever places the observers are located. Thus, for field trials of variability among histopathologists, radiologists, or laboratory chemists, a set of roentgenographic films, tissue slides, or specimens of blood can easily be transported to different institutions, cities, or nations. If the entities under observation are non-preservable transient clinical phenomena, such as the condition of a patient, however, this type of transportation is usually impossible. To study variability, the observers must be assembled at the site where the observed entity occurs. For example, as noted in Chapter 11, a field trial of the Apgar score would require that the observers who rate the newborns' conditions be available at the same birth rooms and be present when each baby is born. Such a trial could be done if we were willing to compare the observations made by different members of the team—such as nurse, obstetrician, and medical student—who are present at the time of each delivery. If we want to compare the same nurse, same obstetrician, and same medical student, however, the difficulty of assembling the same observers for each delivery would make the study unfeasible.

This type of problem can be avoided if the field trial is aimed at a secondary activity—the work done at a later stage of the clinimetric process, after the primary observations are completed, when the observed data are converted into an index. Thus, we could send the observers a descriptive account of a newborn baby's heart rate, respiratory rate, physical appearance and responses, and then invite the observers to transform this information into an Apgar score. Very few clinicians, however, would be satisfied that this type of secondary conversion of data would be an adequate investigation of observer variability in use of the Apgar index.

On the other hand, the secondary transformation of basic data can sometimes be an important phenomenon that justifies separate field trials. For example, national and international data on vital statistics depend on the selection of a single cause of death from the various diagnoses and other information listed on a death certificate. Despite various coding manuals, "nosology guidelines," and other forms of instruction, this clinimetric task can be performed with major variability by coding clerks in different nations. The discovery of an unacceptably high degree of inconsistency in this process[31] was one of many factors that have led to substantial doubts about the scientific quality of international data for "vital statistics."[54]

Similar types of disagreement in secondary observational decisions may occur when different clinical judges are given a summary of a patient's medical record, rather than the actual record itself, and are asked to decide the cause of the patient's death. The variability noted in these secondary decisions can be a fertile source of controversy for both the classification of outcome events and the subsequent statistical conclusions of randomized clinical trials (or other forms of research).

13.2.2. STUDIES OF VALIDITY

The purpose and setting of the index will affect the decision to examine criterion validity, construct validity, or both in a field trial. As discussed in Chapter 12, certain clinimetric indexes can be tested against a definitive gold-standard criterion; others may be tested against an accepted cognate substitute; and all will require validation by application to show whether the index is clinically worthwhile. Since the design of these trials will be discussed in Section 13.3, the rest of this section is concerned with two additional types of validation that commonly occur in clinimetric work.

13.2.2.1. *Critical Comparisons*

When a new index is developed, the investigator will often want to show its superiority to existing indexes that measure the same or an analogous phenomenon. These demonstrations usually involve a head-on-head comparison in which the results of the new index are directly contrasted with those of the old one. The goal may be to show the distinctive dissociations described in Section 12.3.4.2, but the trial can also have several other purposes.

In one instance, the trial may be intended to show that the new index is quicker, easier, and cheaper to use than the previous index while producing essentially similar results. In another instance, the goal may be to show that the new index can be used with less observer variability or with higher scores for criterion validity than the old one.

Although distinctive dissociations can be shown with an appropriate statistical coefficient, many clinical scientists would want to see direct evidence and not just a correlation coefficient. This evidence can be presented in the form of a table or graph that shows the simultaneous agreements and disagreements in values for the two indexes. Alternatively, if the indexes are applied to an external variable, their impact on the external variable can be evaluated. For example, for use as a diagnostic marker, we might check whether new index A is alone more accurate than old index B, or whether the results of index B, when supplemented by those of index A, become diagnostically improved. If the two indexes are both used for prognostic predictions, the two can be compared in conjoint strata, searching for the gradients-within-gradients phenomenon described in Section 4.3.2.3. The existence of these double-gradients would show that the new index has prognostic effects not demarcated by the old index.

Samet[140] has written a perceptive commentary about the need for this type of direct comparison in questionnaires dealing with respiratory symptoms; and an excellent example of the process was later provided when Comstock et al.[17] contrasted a new and old questionnaire on respiratory symptoms.

13.2.2.2. *Confirmation Challenges in New Groups*

A type of validation that is increasingly sought for clinimetric indexes is to test its performance in a new group of people, different from the ones in whom the index was originally developed. The index may have shown good statistical results when tested for consistency and validity in the set of people in whom it was developed. This set is often called the *training, developmental,* or *generating* set. For the additional new confirmation of validity, the index is then tested in a different set of people—the *challenge* or *test* set.

This new set of people can be a different group of presumably similar patients assembled later at the same institution, or similar patients assembled elsewhere. There are two main reasons for this additional form of validation. The first is that the pilot studies and other activities conducted during the developmental process may have led to various ad hoc adjustments that made the index too custom-tailored for the immediate clinical group under study. When applied in some other clinical situation, the index might not work as well.

The second reason is that the index may have been produced by a mathematical model in which certain variables became important not because of their biologic cogency but because of numerical caprices in the variances calculated from the data. The flaws of an index constructed in this mainly mathematical manner may not become evident until the index is checked in some other group of patients. For example, when a multivariate mathematical model was used to construct an index that predicted whether emergency-room patients with chest pain had acute myocardial infarction,[69] the index did not perform well when tested later at another institution.[28] The problem was believed to be statistical, arising because the second group of patients had a prevalence of myocardial infarction different from that of the first group.

13.3. **Structure of the Trial**

The basic structure of a field trial can be described according to the architectural model used for any form of process research.[54] In the type of field trial under consideration here, the process leads to the results that emerge when the index is used. Investigations of the process are concerned with agreement between observers (for tests of consistency), between the index and a selected standard (for tests of criterion validity), or between the index and some other non-standard index (for testing distinctiveness in construct validity).

When construct validity is checked in a specific application of the index, the research is seldom regarded as a field trial and the investigative structure depends on the type of application. For example, a new index of pain might have its construct validity demonstrated by its ability to discriminate active treatment from placebo in a randomized trial of the two agents. Such research would be regarded mainly as a study of therapy, not as a field trial of the index.

As exercises in process research, field trials of consistency or validity can be analyzed using the structure of an architectural model, which is outlined with an *input* receiving a *procedure* that leads to an *output*.[54] To evaluate the research, we consider the appropriate suitability and comparable similarity of each of the main structural components—input, procedures, and output. Because the output scales of clinimetric indexes usually receive substantial attention before a field trial is reached, the input and procedures are the main topics to be considered when the trial is planned and evaluated.

13.3.1. SUITABILITY OF INPUT

The input in a field trial consists of the particular groups of patients, specimens, or other entities that are being rated with the index. To be suitable, the groups should contain both a broad and a representative spectrum of challenges.

13.3.1.1. *Broad Spectrum*

An index will not be effectively tested if the groups under study do not contain an adequately broad spectrum of challenges. For example, an index concerned with rating functional disability might show fallaciously excellent consistency and validity if most of the patients under study are relatively normal, without any substantial impairments in function.

13.3.1.2. *Representative Spectrum*

Another source of inadequate testing is a spectrum that does not suitably represent the groups to whom the index will later be applied. For example, many diagnostic-marker indexes are tested in hospital populations selected to contain roughly equal numbers of diseased and non-diseased patients. Because this type of spectrum does not represent the world outside the hospital, the index will usually have erroneously elevated values of "predictive accuracy," thus leading to major disappointments when the index is later used for screening purposes in the lower prevalence of the disease found in a more general population.[54]

The challenges of broad scope and adequate representativeness can seldom be satisfied with a single group. If the group is adequately representative, it may not include some of the uncommon conditions needed for extensive scope; and if scope is extensive, the selected group may not be representative. Consequently, a suitable test process often requires a combination of two groups: one chosen for scope and the other for representativeness. Thus, a diagnostic marker index might be tested in an unselected representative group containing a large number of consecutive patients. To augment the scope of the group, it would be enlarged to include patients specifically chosen to have the uncommon conditions that would encompass a wider spectrum of disease and control patients.

13.3.1.3. *Subgroup Analysis*

Beyond these issues in spectrum, a suitable *subgroup analysis* is usually needed to show that an index is pertinent for its proposed clinical setting. For such an analysis, the results of an index are shown in subgroups of patients stratified according to the clinical conditions that will be of greatest interest when subsequent users employ the index. For example, clinicians might want to know whether a diagnostic marker index has the same sensitivity and specificity for patients with mild disease or severe disease, with or without symptoms, and with or without certain forms of co-morbidity. This type of information would require a suitable stratification, showing the results in the appropriate subgroups.

13.3.2. SIMILARITY OF INPUT

To get a fair comparison of two indexes (or two performances of the same index) the input submitted to the index should be essentially similar on both occasions. This distinction may be overlooked in at least three types of situation that produce inappropriate or biased comparisons. The observed phenomenon may be unstable; the results of one index may affect the choice of people exposed to the second; or the indexes may be compared in the disparate groups of different clinical settings.

13.3.2.1. *Unstable Phenomena*

Measurements of the same phenomenon can disagree if the phenomenon itself changes during the interval between measurements. For example, a person's basic clinical condition may have been altered; or an individual variable, such as blood pressure or weight, may undergo regular fluctuations in a diurnal or other cycle of periodicity. If these additional sources of change are not properly considered, the observed variability may be incorrectly attributed to the mensuration process.

In studies of *inter*-observer variability, this problem can often be avoided by arranging for only a very short time to elapse between the examinations performed by the two (or more) observers whose agreement is being tested. On the other hand, because the individual observers will recall their previous ratings, a short interval cannot be used between the repeated examinations used to test *intra*-observer variability. Consequently, for many indexes that require subjective appraisal of a patient's clinical condition, inter-observer variability becomes the only feasible method of testing for consistency.

13.3.2.2. *Sequential-Ordering Bias*

A different type of problem occurs if the group chosen to be exposed to the second index is affected by the results found with the first index. For indexes used as diagnostic markers, this problem has been called "work-up bias" or "sequential ordering bias."[54,135] It arises if the result of the marker index is used to decide whether and when to compare it against a cognate index or against a definitive diagnostic test. When the results of the two sets of indexes are later compared, the comparison will be distorted by the selection process. For example, in asymptomatic middle-aged men, coronary arteriography will often be ordered if an exercise stress test is positive, but not if the stress test is negative. By selectively adding patients with positive stress tests to the total group, this work-up bias will enrich the proportions of patients who have true positive and false positive results. The consequence of the distorted spectrum of challenges will be a falsely high sensitivity and a falsely low specificity for the stress test as a diagnostic marker of coronary artery disease.

13.3.2.3. *Changes in Clinical Setting*

The type of confirmation challenge discussed in Section 13.2.2.2 can serve two roles. Its most obvious function is to demonstrate the validity of the index in a group of people different from the group in which the index was developed. In this type of challenge, the two groups should contain different people but should have similar clinical conditions and frameworks. If the clinical conditions or frameworks have been substantially altered, disagreements arising from the changed situations may be incorrectly attributed to flaws in the index.

For example, suppose an index has been developed to diagnose the likelihood of pneumonia in patients who appear with fever and cough at the emergency room of a large municipal hospital. When checked in a confirmation challenge, the index may show impaired validity if the new clinical group under study is located at a Veterans Hospital, small community hospital, or other circumstances where patterns of self-referral by patients or iatric referral by physicians may greatly alter the disease spectrum of the fever and cough under examination.

The latter situation demonstrates a second important role for confirmation challenges. They may sometimes be deliberately constructed to demonstrate the inadequacy of an index rather than to verify its success. For example, if the diagnostic index for pneumonia has been well constructed biologically, it should not be affected by the spectrum of fever and cough. The index should be able to deal appropriately with patients having different forms of these two symptoms, regardless of the relative frequency of their pattern in the spectrum of patients under examination. If a change in this relative frequency affects the performance of the index, its original construction may have been excessively dependent on statistical rather than biologic attributes of the patients under study. Because the challenge procedure would demonstrate the defective performance of the index in a different clinical spectrum, someone who suspects the existence of such defects might deliberately choose an altered spectrum to show the problems.

13.3.3. SUITABILITY OF PROCEDURES

For an index to be adequately tested, its operating procedure must be carried out properly. For example, a laboratory measurement would not be properly conducted if the chemical reagents have the wrong concentration or if the spectrophotometer receives the wrong electrical voltage. In clinimetric indexes, the procedure may be flawed because of problems in the site where an examination is done (e.g., auscultation in a noisy room vs. a quiet room;

inspection of cyanosis or jaundice in a room with unsuitable lighting or background colors), or because of unrecognized variations in the way the process is performed. For example, certain terms that facilitate satisfactory response to oral questions might be better explained to patients by one set of examiners than by another set. The different results noted for the index in these two sets of circumstances might then be ascribed erroneously to factors inherent in the observation process rather than to differences in clarity of explanation.

13.3.4. SIMILARITY OF PROCEDURES

In the example just cited, the difference in procedures would have led to an erroneous conclusion. Unless suitable precautions are taken in other circumstances, a biased comparison of two indexes may lead to falsely high or low results for consistency and validity. This type of bias can arise if suitable blinding is not used to maintain objectivity in the compared observations. Observer bias, which can occur overtly or inadvertently, is well illustrated by problems in the testing of indexes used as diagnostic markers.

For example, when the nitro-blue tetrazolium (NBT) test was used in diagnosis of bacterial infection, the sensitivity originally reported for the new test was sharply reduced when the subjective interpretations of the test were performed by observers who were unaware of the correct diagnosis.[135] In other diagnostic circumstances, such as exercise stress testing and coronary arteriography, an observer interpreting the arteriogram in ordinary clinical practice usually knows the results of the stress test. Unless the arteriograms are reinterpreted objectively, a study of the diagnostic sensitivity and specificity of the exercise stress test may yield falsely high results.

Certain field trials may be intended to show the inadvertent bias produced by an observer's knowledge of ancillary clinical data. Thus, a group of radiologists substantially altered their interpretation of sequential chest films in a set of patients when the same films for each patient were submitted in a random order, out of the natural clinical sequence.[136]

13.4. **Problems in Interpreting Field Trials**

The development of a new clinimetric index can be likened to the phases used in the development of a new drug. In Phase I, the index is conceived and created. In Phase II, the index is evaluated for sensibility and tested with various pilot studies. In Phase III, the index receives field trials that demonstrate the consistency and validity it acquired during the preceding phases. Most indexes are generally reported (or "marketed") at this point in their development, although many important indexes—such as the original TNM staging systems for cancer and the Jones diagnostic criteria for rheumatic fever—have come into usage without any accompanying evidence from field trials. The confirmation of the index in new test groups (as discussed in Section 13.2.2.2) will then serve as a counterpart of Phase IV in drug development.

If the index has been properly developed and if it received a suitable pre-trial evaluation and an appropriately planned field trial, the trial should produce worthwhile scientific data. If these issues have not been well managed, the trial can create new problems. The most prominent problems, which are discussed in the next three subsections, arise from false negative or false positive results in poorly planned trials or from trials that are overinterpreted.

13.4.1. FALSE NEGATIVE RESULTS

A good index may be deemed poor because of low statistical values for consistency or validity. This type of false negative result is most likely to arise if the field trial is done prematurely before the index has been suitably improved with pilot studies, but the problem can also occur if the field trial is constructed without adequate attention to the features of suitability and similarity noted throughout Section 13.3. For example, a diagnostic index that works well when applied to the data available at the time of a patient's discharge from the hospital may not work well if applied in a field trial for patients newly admitted to the hospital. Instead of recognizing that the setting of the field trial had been altered, the investigators may conclude that the index is unsatisfactory.

13.4.2. FALSE POSITIVE RESULTS

The converse of the situation just cited occurs when an unsatisfactory index gets good results in a field trial. This problem is particularly likely to arise when an important issue in biased observation—as noted in Section 13.3.4—has been overlooked. The problem can also occur, however, in a field trial that is large enough to produce impressive stochastic results for statistical significance, even though the descriptive statistics show relatively unimpressive values.[54]

13.4.3. OVER-INTERPRETATION

The main false positive hazard in field trials, however, occurs when an index is accepted as satisfactory merely because it had high values of consistency and validity. If these high values obscure or eliminate an evaluation of sensibility, an inadequate index may become widely promulgated before its inherent defects are recognized.

This problem commonly occurs when investigators seek an index to use in a new research project. Because the investigators are concerned with the particular intervention or hypothesis that is being appraised in the research, they will usually concentrate their energies on this aspect of the appraisal. Because the index will serve "merely" as a source of data, the investigators will prefer not to develop a new index, and will usually look for something that has been previously tested and found to be "reliable" and "valid." Unless the investigators carefully interpret the field trial that produced the coefficients of reliability and validity, however, the existing index may turn out to be unsatisfactory for its new purpose. The field trial may have been conducted with an input and procedures that were drastically different from the circumstances in which the investigators now propose to use the index.

The problem has become particularly striking as functional capacity and quality of life become increasingly evaluated as part of randomized trials of medical, surgical, or psychosocial interventions.[61] When the trial is over, the investigators may sometimes find that they failed to learn what they really wanted to know. The index they used was reliable and valid according to the results of its previous field trials, but it was unsuitable for the specific goals of the new research. The index may have been insensitive to change, aimed at the wrong focus, intended for different patients observed in different clinical settings, or otherwise inadequate for its newly assigned role.

The problem can be avoided if investigators recognize that statistical coefficients should not be accepted without an evaluation of the study from which they emanated. In many instances, the construction of an appropriate new index—although an unappealing extra burden in the research—may ultimately be less costly in time and effort than the naive usage of a validated index that works improperly. Besides, if the investigators concentrate on a suitable focus and sensibility for the new index, its development and testing may not require the mammoth efforts that are sometimes expended in a ritualistic approach to field trials.

Chapter 14

A Pragmatic Taxonomy for Classifying Clinimetric Indexes

All the discussion so far has been concerned with the strategies used to construct clinical indexes and to evaluate their accomplishments. The strategies can be applied for any individual index, but sometimes we may want to compare the members of a group of relatively similar indexes. In such a comparison, the goal might be to choose which index is best for use in a particular situation or to determine whether new indexes should be developed. To do those comparative evaluations, we need a method of classifying indexes into groups that are similar enough to warrant a distinction of their differences. If several indexes are too disparate from one another, an effort to compare them would be pointless—somewhat like contrasting apples, oranges, and grapes—but if the indexes are reasonably similar, an attempt to distinguish among them can be important and worthwhile, particularly if we want to choose one of them for future usage.

For example, suppose we want to evaluate indexes that describe the clinical severity of a particular disease. If we assemble individual indexes for the clinical severity of such diseases as myocardial infarction, chronic pulmonary disease, cancer of the colon, or renal failure, we can evaluate each index separately, but the group of indexes might be too diverse for the individual members to be compared against one another. If the indexes of clinical severity all refer to the same type of disease, such as cancer, a description of severity for cancers in the lung, breast, colon, or prostate might still be too disease-specific for the indexes to be individually compared, although certain common attributes might be excerpted for inclusion in a new index of "clinical severity in cancer." On the other hand, a more general set of indexes of clinical severity—based on symptoms, physiologic abnormalities, or other attributes that are not disease-specific—might be quite suitable for direct comparison and evaluation.

To allow clinimetric indexes to be compared, we therefore need a way of classifying them into reasonably similar groups. The purpose of this chapter is to develop a pragmatic taxonomy for those classifications. The taxonomy is intended as a catalog that puts appropriate indexes in the same categorical group, within which they can then be evaluated for their differences. The categories should act as a mechanism that can help both in classifying the available indexes and in identifying problems whose solutions can lead to new, improved indexes.

For a classification to be derived from pragmatic reality, the first step is to collect a series of diverse indexes that become the taxonomic challenge. Section 14.1 contains an account of the methods by which my colleagues and I assembled several thousand publications that were reviewed during our taxonomic activities. The sections that follow thereafter will present the proposed system of classification.

14.1. Assembly and Selection of Clinical Indexes

Because clinical indexes have received so little attention as a distinct investigative entity in clinical science, they can seldom be located with the customary procedures used to find things in the medical literature. My main source of information about clinical indexes has been a large file, deliberately collected during the past two decades, of reprints, tear sheets, replicated material, three-by-five cards, or other references to publications in medical literature. The material has been catalogued under such major headings as *Clinical Trials, Indexes, Scales, Predictors, Prognosis, Natural History*, and *Course.* Each of these headings has usually had a subheading indicating a particular organ system. Thus, indexes for peptic ulcer disease could be found, with gastrointestinal (GI) subheadings, as part of the collections marked *Clin. Trials, GI; Indexes, GI; Predictors, GI;* etc. Similarly, indexes for congestive heart failure or coronary heart disease were found in analogous headings that had the subtitles of *cardiac* or *coronary*.

This collection of reprint material served as a starting point for identifying clinical indexes in a particular topic. The references cited in the original articles would often identify other sources, which were then pursued in a branching pattern of expansion until all the main leads seemed to have been covered.

To choose the indexes that were going to be classified, we defined a clinimetric index as a variable, containing clinical data, that had received distinct analytic attention in a published report. Several types of evidence were regarded as showing distinct analytic attention. The index might have offered the criteria that circumscribed the patients admitted to or excluded from a particular study. The index could provide data that were quantitatively summarized in the results or that were displayed in tables or graphs. If the investigators stated that certain information had been collected in the research, but if the information was not used in circumscriptions, tabulations, summaries, graphs, or other formal analyses, the information was not regarded as representing an index in that study.

An index was deemed to contain clinical data if its component variables included patients' symptoms, physical findings, or certain forms of data (such as diagnoses or prognoses) produced by clinical reasoning. Indexes that contained only paraclinical data—from morphologic or laboratory evidence—were not included. For example, indexes that reflect decisions based exclusively on electrolyte abnormalities, electrocardiographic patterns, differentiation of cancer cells, or radiographic occlusion of coronary arteries were regarded as paraclinical. If paraclinical information was combined with clinical data (for diagnostic or other decisions), the index was classified as clinical.

14.2. Problems in Classification by Topic

Before my colleagues and I started assembling the cited material, we thought the work would be relatively easy. All that seemed necessary was to collect reports of all the indexes dealing with a particular clinical entity (such as peptic ulcer, rheumatoid arthritis, or coronary disease) and then to divide the indexes topically according to their functional roles in denoting status, change, prognosis, or guidelines for that entity. We soon found that this expectation was much too simplistic.

The first problem came with the discovery that so many indexes were out there. We had expected to find two-digit numbers: perhaps 10 or 20 indexes for each entity, but surely no more than 100. Instead, we found three-digit figures: often more than several hundred indexes had been used in various formats and contents for the entities under consideration.

A second problem was that the investigators using a particular index often seemed unaware of other options. Their index had been chosen or developed without any stated reasons for the process: alternative existing indexes were seldom mentioned, compared, or appraised. Consequently, if we wanted to annotate our compendium by referring to the evaluations that had been done for each index, we seldom found any evaluations to work with. We could use our own qualitative criteria (see Chapter 10) to try to assess things such as sensibility, but we would seldom be able to cite quantitative data for tests of consistency or validity.

The third problem was particularly striking. It arose from the enormous diversity of the indexes, especially those used to describe status. In creating indexes, the investigators had focused on a vast array of different distinctions—alone or in combination—for each entity under consideration. To arrange those diverse indexes into an orderly compendium would require the development of much more specific categories than the basic division of status, change, prediction, and guideline. Although satisfactory as major groupings, these terms would need many subdivisions to be suitable for the taxonomic task of a compendium. The next few sections contain an account of the taxonomies developed for this purpose.

14.3. General Principles of Classification

We wanted a system that would assign each index to a particular clinical condition and that would assign that condition topographically to a particular part of the body. Although topographically oriented, however, the classification scheme would also have to encompass indexes that might be pertinent for several or many diseases.

For example, an index for the severity of delayed post-prandial pain, relieved by alkali or food, refers to a type of distress usually associated with peptic ulcer; and the index could not readily be applied to many diseases other than peptic ulcer. On the other hand, an index that rates the severity of nausea, vomiting, diarrhea, or constipation might be pertinent for patients with peptic ulcer, but could also be used for many other gastrointestinal ailments. An index that expresses a patient's state of health as generally well or sick, or an index of general functional state (referring to attributes such as occupational capacity or activities of daily living) could be applied to a broad range of clinical conditions.

To deal with this diversity, we developed mechanisms to catalog clinical ailments according to pathologic and topographic levels of their associated phenomena, and to identify different parts of the clinical spectrum of a disease.

14.3.1. PATHOLOGIC LEVELS OF DISEASE PHENOMENA

In etiologic and pathophysiologic reasoning, the phenomena of disease extend upward from inciting agents (such as microbial organisms) to inflamed tissue (such as pneumonitis) to gross disorders (such as disruption of blood vessels) to clinical manifestations (such as coughing blood). In diagnostic reasoning, the phenomena are often analyzed in a downward direction from gross clinical manifestations (such as difficulty in swallowing) that are explicated by gross disorders (such as esophageal obstruction) that are further explicated by patho-anatomic disease entities (such as esophageal cancer).[44]

This three-tier level of pathologic classification will suffice for most clinimetric purposes. A clinimetric index may deal with the overt clinical manifestations that constitute symptoms and physical signs; with other phenomena that represent gross pathophysiologic disorders (such as obstruction, reflux, or decompensation); or with the discrete etiologic or patho-anatomic entities that are often called diseases.

14.3.2. TOPOGRAPHIC LEVELS OF DISEASE PHENOMENA

The topographic sites of clinimetric phenomena can be classified by dividing the body into a series of *domains*.[44] A domain can be an individual organ (such as the heart or liver), a region (such as the chest or abdomen), a channel (such as the gastrointestinal or urinary tract), or a system (such as the cardiopulmonary system, endocrine glands, hematopoietic apparatus, or body as a whole).

The domain concept is particularly useful in the explanatory processes of diagnostic reasoning, but it also allows a topographic categorization for diseases (such as leukemia, inflammatory bowel disease, or hypopituitarism) whose effects cannot always be localized to a single anatomic structure. The domain concept also allows a more detailed definition of a *disorder*, which is a gross abnormality in the structure or function of a domain. The abnormality can involve the size, composition, or location of a structural lesion, or the quantitative amount, operation, or direction of a dysfunction.[44] Thus, gastrointestinal obstruction or perforation, and cardiac arrhythmias or decompensation, would be classified as disorders. Disorders are also cited in such terms as hypertrophy or atrophy, -megaly, distention, reflux, hyper- or hypo-perfusion, irritation (as in irritable bowel syndrome), and overproduction or underproduction (e.g., hyper- or hypo-thyroidism).

A single clinical manifestation, such as dyspnea, can be due to several possible disorders, such as respiratory failure or cardiac decompensation, each of which can be due to many possible patho-anatomic or etiologic entities of disease.

14.3.3. THE CLINICAL SPECTRUM OF DISEASE

Each disease or ailment has a spectrum of possible phenomena, which can involve different clinical attributes. The attributes include the type of manifestations, the timing of manifestations, the co-morbidity of concomitant additional ailments, and such ancillary features as therapeutic agents and sociopersonal status.

14.3.3.1. *Types of Manifestations*

A particular disease entity can sometimes be clinically "silent," producing no overt symptoms or other clinical manifestations. In many other instances, however, the disease produces primary manifestations, secondary manifestations, or both.[38]

Primary manifestations are attributable to the main or characteristic "lesion" of the disease. For example, the characteristic pains of peptic ulcer, coronary artery disease, or rheumatoid arthritis arise respectively from the basic lesion or dysfunction in the stomach or duodenum, anoxemic myocardium, or affected joints. *Secondary* manifestations arise as the disease produces gross disorders, complications, spread, or systemic effects. The secondary manifestations can occur specifically in the original topographic site of the disease; they can occur at other topographic sites; or they can involve a more *systemic* reaction in the body as a whole. For example, bleeding or vomiting might be secondary gastrointestinal complications of peptic ulcer, but weight loss would be a systemic effect. In coronary artery disease, angina pectoris would be a primary manifestation, arrhythmias or congestive heart failure would be secondary cardiac disorders, and fatigue or incapacitation would be systemic effects. The effects that arise as systemic manifestations (such as weight loss or fatigue) are often separated from the clinically focal disorders that may be regarded as complications. Thus, in the spectrum of patients with coronary disease, weight loss or fatigue would be classified as a systemic effect, whereas arrhythmias or congestive failure would be cited as secondary complications.

The distinctions of primary, systemic, and secondary manifestations have sometimes been used in attempts to distinguish illness from disease. Thus, if a *disease* is a morphologic, biochemical, or microbiologic entity observed in tissues, cells, fluids, or microscopic specimens, an *illness* consists of the primary, secondary, or systemic clinical manifestations that occur directly in the patient. Not all disease produces illness: certain diseases are detected while they are clinically silent and symptomless. Conversely, not all illness is due to disease: many aspects of fatigue, disability, dysfunction, or other human distresses arise from psychic or social factors that may not be regarded as "disease."

The secondary manifestations of a disease are seldom unique to that disease and can usually be produced by many other ailments. Thus, bleeding or vomiting can arise from diverse gastrointestinal diseases other than peptic ulcer; arrhythmias or congestive heart failure can be caused by many cardiac ailments other than coronary disease; and weight loss, fatigue, or incapacitation can arise from diverse diseases or problems that are neither gastrointestinal nor cardiac.

14.3.3.2.   *Additional Attributes*

Although the primary, systemic and/or secondary manifestations help identify patients in different parts of the spectrum of a particular disease, several other attributes can create further differentiation of the spectrum. The attributes include the timing of manifestations, the co-morbidity of associated diseases, and the ancillary features of therapy and sociopersonal status. These attributes will be further discussed in Sections 14.4.1.4–14.4.1.6.

Since all of the distinctions in types of manifestations, timing of manifestations, co-morbidity, and ancillary features might be needed among indexes used to describe a particular disease, and since some of the indexes might readily be applied for many other diseases or clinical conditions, the clinimetric taxonomy should provide for both the specific details and the broader application of the indexes under consideration.

14.4. Basic Taxonomic Arrangements

The principles cited in Sections 14.3.1–14.3.3 allow the formulation of a general topographic classification for clinimetric indexes. For a particular disease or ailment, the *ailment-oriented* indexes can be cited in six main groups as *ailment-specific, disorder-specific, systemic, temporal, co-morbid,* or *ancillary.* Since all of these indexes refer to components of the spectrum of a particular ailment, a seventh group—called *spectral*—is formed by indexes that contain combinations of two or more entries from the foregoing six groups.

A separate classification is used for the *general* indexes of health or functional state that can be applied to anyone, regardless of a specific disease or ailment. When components from a general index are combined with components from one of the various spectral indexes, the result can be called a *hybrid index.* The taxonomy is further described in the sections that follow.

14.4.1.   AILMENT-ORIENTED INDEXES

The term *ailment-oriented* is used to refer to indexes that refer to diseases, disorders, symptoms, clinical conditions, and other manifestations that are the characteristic focus of attention in clinical care. The ailment-oriented indexes are distinguished from *general* indexes of health status or function that are used without reference to specific clinical manifestations or conditions.

14.4.1.1. *Ailment-Specific Indexes*

The indexes used to diagnose the existence of a particular clinical ailment are specific for that ailment and can be called *ailment-specific*. Such indexes may refer to diagnosis of a disease (such as myocardial infarction), a disorder (such as stroke, congestive heart failure, or gastrointestinal bleeding), or a symptom (such as anorexia).

Indexes that offer graded ratings for the severity or magnitude of a particular ailment are sometimes used in a manner that is specific to that ailment, but they can also be used in studies of other ailments. For example, an index of severity for congestive heart failure would be ailment-specific in a study of treatment for congestive heart failure, but would have a different role in a study of coronary artery disease.

Within the spectrum of symptomatic manifestations for a particular disease, certain indexes might refer to primary manifestations (such as the postprandial pain of peptic ulcer) or to secondary disorders and manifestations (such as obstructive phenomena or weight loss). Some primary manifestations might be further classified as characteristic or principal features of the ailment, whereas other primary manifestations might be less typical. For example, hemoptysis is a characteristic primary feature of lung cancer, but wheezing, when caused by the cancer's obstruction of a bronchial lumen, occurs less frequently.

14.4.1.2. *Disorder-Specific Indexes*

According to their apparent pathogenesis, many of the secondary manifestations of an ailment can be classified as disorder-specific. To avoid invidious decisions about pathogenesis, however, certain manifestations can be arbitrarily classified as either ailment-specific or disorder-specific, without a profound analysis of pathophysiologic distinctions and justifications. For example, the heartburn associated with acid reflux in peptic ulcer could be regarded as either a primary (ailment-specific) or as a secondary (disorder-specific) manifestation. If an index for heartburn in peptic ulcer is arbitrarily classified as *disorder-specific,* the goal is to give the index a taxonomic home rather than to offer judgments about pathophysiologic controversies and uncertainties.

The richness of the taxonomic subdivisions offered under the ailment-specific and disorder-specific titles will depend on the extensiveness of the network of symptoms and other clinical manifestations for whatever entity is under study. In some instances, an ailment-specific index may contain several primary symptoms, a combination of primary and (disorder-specific) secondary symptoms, or other constituents taken from other categories of classification.

14.4.1.3. *Indexes for Systemic Symptoms*

Systemic symptoms—such as anorexia, weight loss, and fatigue—are difficult to classify. When attributable to a specific ailment, such as cancer or congestive heart failure, they can be ascribed to the body as a whole rather than to a more specific pathologic site in an organ, region, channel, or localized system. This type of "holistic" localization, however, does not imply that the disease has had a physical or "organic" spread beyond its primary location or source. Because the systemic phenomena can be produced by psychic effects, such as depression, rather than by "toxins" or other circulated effects of an organic disease, systemic manifestations often require further attention to differentiate their sources. Thus, fatigue can be an important indication of cancer severity if ascribable to the cancer itself, but may not have the same total impact if due to a reversible psychic depression. For analogous reasons, in a society where weight loss is often deliberately sought for cosmetic reasons, the manifestation of weight loss should be differentiated according to its purposeful or non-purposeful provocation.

In some instances, such as the paraneoplastic syndromes associated with certain cancers, the tumor can exercise a distant hormonal effect without having anatomically spread beyond its primary site. Manifestations of this type can also be cited in the systemic category. In other circumstances, an apparently systemic symptom such as anorexia may actually be a primary manifestation of a gastric disease.

For all these reasons, the classification of systemic symptoms will depend on the context in which they occur. In many instances, they will be associated with a particular ailment and included as part of the spectrum of that ailment.

14.4.1.4. *Temporal Attributes*

Regardless of whether a particular manifestation is cited in an ailment-specific, disorder-specific, or systemic category, many clinical phenomena are regularly classified according to features of time. The temporal feature may be cited in terms of *frequency* as **often** or **seldom;** in *duration* as **long** or **short, acute** or **chronic;** in *rate of progression* as **fast** or **slow;** or in other chronometric expressions. The temporal attributes can be cited in this category if they are the sole focus of the index. If the temporal features are combined with other clinical manifestations, the combination can be cited as a *spectral* index (Section 14.4.1.7).

14.4.1.5.   *Indexes of Co-Morbidity*

Because many patients in modern medicine are found to have more than one disease, the identification of whatever is chosen as the "main" ailment must be supplemented with attention to the effects of the other coexisting diseases. In some instances, the co-morbid disease may be trivial, such as a small ocular cataract that has no effect on the status of someone with coronary disease. On the other hand, a co-morbid ailment may have a major impact on the patient's total severity of illness. For example, suppose two patients are both found to have an asymptomatic **Stage I** cancer. One of the patients may be in excellent health and have an excellent prognosis, whereas the other may die shortly afterward because of severe co-morbid disease in the heart, lungs, or elsewhere. This major difference in the patients would be unidentified and unrecognized if they were both classified merely as being in the asymptomatic **Stage I** of the clinical spectrum of the cancer.

14.4.1.6.   *Ancillary Indexes*

The severity or other attributes of a clinical condition are sometimes described according to phenomena used in the care of that condition. For example, the severity of angina pectoris might be rated according to the number of ancillary nitroglycerine tablets consumed by the patient each week. Similarly, severity might be rated according to supplemental antacid treatment for peptic ulcer, or bronchodilator inhalants for chronic pulmonary disease.

Although greatly appealing because the amount of ancillary therapy can be readily quantified, these indexes have two main hazards. The first is that "severity," being dependent on the patient's decision to take (or a doctor's decision to give) additional treatment, becomes a highly subjective phenomenon, with no actual rating given or attempted for the magnitude of the severity itself. A second problem is that the ancillary treatment can be taken for prophylactic or remedial purposes, or both. Thus, certain patients may use nitroglycerin, antacids, or bronchodilator inhalants prophylactically before undertaking an act that might evoke symptoms, whereas other patients may use the medication only in a remedial manner after appropriate symptoms have appeared. If no distinctions are made between prophylactic and remedial use of medication, its quantity can be greatly misleading as an index of the magnitude of severity. A highly anxious patient, for example, might consume a great deal of prophylactic medication to avoid symptoms that might not occur even if the medication were not used. A therapy-based ancillary index should therefore contain arrangements to separate prophylactic vs. remedial uses of the therapy and to determine the kinds of stimuli that have evoked the therapy.

Another type of ancillary index depends on sociopersonal attributes of the patient. Such indexes are used when the spectrum of an ailment is cited according to age, gender, family background, occupation, or socioeconomic status. The ancillary indexes may also include such psychic or behavioral attributes as stress, anxiety, or personality type.

14.4.1.7. *Spectral Indexes*

Spectral indexes contain mixtures of several individual manifestations from the primary, secondary, systemic, temporal, co-morbid, or ancillary features in the spectrum of a particular ailment. For example, in a spectral index for peptic ulcer, the patient could receive a rating that depends on a combination of pain as a primary feature, constipation as a secondary feature, weight loss as a systemic feature, frequency of pain as a temporal feature, and chronic lung disease as a co-morbid feature. Since all five of these manifestations are part of the spectrum of clinical phenomena associated with peptic ulcer, their combination can be regarded as a *spectral index.* If the combination is expanded to include "external" components referring to general health or functional status, the result could be regarded as a *hybrid index.*

In many indexes of clinical condition—such as the Apgar Score for the status of a newborn baby—several different manifestations are combined into a single rating. The name given to such indexes is optional. They can be called *spectral* or *composite,* according to the preference of the user. (My own preference is to call them *composite* and to reserve *spectral* for circumstances dealing with a particular disease and its associated spectrum.)

In certain circumstances, analogous to those of diagnostic marker tests, a spectral index is used to identify a part of the spectrum of a disease. For example, the carcinoembryonic antigen (CEA) has been used as a spectral-marker test to distinguish between localized and metastatic cancer. *Spectral marker indexes* can be classified in the category of spectral indexes. The procedure used to show the accuracy of a spectral index is analogous to the procedure used for validation of diagnostic marker tests.[54]

14.4.2. GENERAL INDEXES

Except for the occasional inclusion of the systemic manifestations discussed in Section 14.4.1.3, general indexes can be divided into two broad categories, dealing with general health and general function.

14.4.2.1. *General Health*

The answer to the classical question "How are you?" produces an index of general health or well-being. Indexes of this type are often quite simple, being cited with a single global rating, but they can become much more complex, particularly if attempts are made to identify the diverse components that may contribute to general health or well-being.

The topic has received major attention during the past decade, and a large variety of complex indexes have been developed to describe health status, life situation, quality of life, and other general features of a person's health or life. The general-health indexes may or may not include specific attention to the functional-state attributes discussed in the next subsection.

14.4.2.2. *Functional State*

Indexes of general function are extraordinarily complicated. They can differ substantially in purpose, scope, setting, contents, construction, and interpretation. In purpose, some indexes are intended as profiles that offer pure description somewhat like a battery of laboratory tests, whereas others are deliberately aggregated into a composite rating that can be summarized and analyzed for groups of people. In scope, the functional states can be physical, emotional, social, or mixtures of these three attributes; and the physical states can refer to basic activities of daily living (such as personal hygiene and mobility), more elaborate activities (such as hobbies and ability to travel), occupational capacity, or mixtures of the foregoing.

Furthermore, some functional-state indexes are relatively ailment-oriented in attempting to restrict themselves to functional problems attributable to the ailment under consideration, whereas other indexes do not attempt to make this pathogenetic distinction. Thus, an index of functional capacity can refer to limitations in physical activity, regardless of their source, or only to those limitations attributable to a particular ailment, such as cardiac disease. An index of occupational capacity might either indicate merely that the patient is unable to work or might note that the inability is due to problems in lungs, heart, extremities, psyche, or national economy.

In setting, the patients under consideration can range from autonomous ambulatory life at home to a bedridden existence in an institution. The contents of the indexes can include relatively few principal questions and variables, or a large number of entities covering a hundred or more items. In construction, the contents can be aggregated with a simple additive score or with an elaborately structured mathematical arrangement.

Regardless of how simple or complicated the functional-state indexes may be, all of them are difficult to interpret for reasons cited earlier in Chapter 6. Most of the indexes do not include attention to patient's preference as a mechanism for selecting important items, and almost all of the indexes ignore the role of patient collaboration. Thus, although functional-status indexes usually depend on ratings for the magnitude of tasks that a patient can perform, attention is seldom given to the concomitant role of the patient's effort and motivation in doing the task, and to the crucial impact of psychic state and social support when pertinent to the performance.[61]

For all these reasons, the classification of functional-state indexes may sometimes differ for each ailment, although the same functional-state indexes may often be used for several different ailments.

14.4.3. HYBRID INDEXES

The word *hybrid* can be used for many different purposes. In this instance, it refers to a mixture in which an index of clinical spectrum—of any of the types noted throughout Sections 14.4.1 and 14.4.2—has been combined with an index of general health or functional status. The term *hybrid* can also be used for indexes containing mixtures of clinical and paraclinical information. For example, many indexes of "disease activity" in rheumatoid arthritis contain hybrid mixtures of spectral, general, and paraclinical data.

14.5. Additional Taxonomic Issues

Section 14.4 offers a catalog for classifying indexes according to the type of clinical condition to which they refer. Within these basic topographic locations, additional classifications can be used for separate problems that can arise from the structure of the indexes or from diverse aspects of their functional roles in describing status, change, predictions, or guidelines.

14.5.1. MANAGEMENT OF GLOBAL SCALES

The global indexes discussed in Chapter 7 will regularly produce two types of problem that can be managed as described in the next two subsections.

14.5.1.1. *Scope of Non-Specific Global Scales*

The characteristic feature of a global scale is the absence of operational criteria to demarcate the output categories. The scale may be presented with such ratings as **0, 1, 2, 3,** or **mild, moderate, severe,** or in the visual analog form of

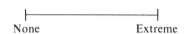

but no further stipulations are provided for decisions in choosing a category or marking the line. In contrast, a demarcated scale might have the same format or set of categories available for selection, but specific directions are provided for each selection.

Because global scales are so easy to construct, they can readily be applied to many different attributes. The same array of global categories or the same visual analog scale might be used separately to rate a broad scope of individual phenomena such as pain, nausea, dyspnea, diarrhea, frequency of distress, problems in sleeping, disability, or dissatisfaction. In other instances, an even simpler global scale, denoted as **present/absent** or **yes/no,** might be used to denote the existence of diverse entities, which thereby become diagnosed without specific criteria being offered for the diagnosis. Global scales of this type are commonly used in checklists for the antecedent presence or absence of such entities as myocardial infarction, pneumonia, chest pain, gastro-intestinal bleeding, use of aspirin, exposure to chemical toxins, etc.

If the same non-specific global scale were applied to a broad scope of entities, and if the scale became repeatedly listed under the indexes available for each of those entities, the list would become excessively long, with relatively little useful information added to compensate for the length. Accordingly, a separate category of non-topographic classification can be used to cite all the non-specific global indexes that have been applied in studies of the main ailment under consideration. The subsequent topographic classifications can then be confined, if so desired, to indexes expressed in demarcated scales.

14.5.1.2. *Aggregated Global Scales*

A different type of taxonomic problem arises when a series of values from global scales are aggregated into a single output rating. For example, a set of successive daily global ratings for pain might be added together to form a weekly pain score; individual global ratings for severity of involvement in different joints might be added to form a total-joint-severity score; individual global ratings for heartburn, nausea, bloating, and waterbrash might be combined to form a dyspepsia score.

If the aggregation process is suitably specified—usually as a simple addition of the individual global values—the rating that appears in the output scale is no longer strictly global. It is clearly demarcated as a sum of the component elements, although the component elements are themselves global. Should this type of aggregation be regarded as a demarcated scale or is it merely a gentrified global rating?

Regardless of how this question is answered, individual global ratings are often aggregated to form output scales that are commonly used and well accepted as measurements in both psychosocial and clinical activities. Aggregates of items that receive global ratings are commonly used as the source of output for most psychosocial indexes, in many of the general clinical indexes used for health and functional status, and in written examinations that test the clinical competence of candidates for licensure or board certification. Accordingly, because aggregated global indexes are so often regarded as demarcated scales, they can be listed among other composite indexes that may have been more fully demarcated.

14.5.2. PROBLEMS IN STATUS INDEXES

Status indexes can create problems in classification if they refer to outcomes (rather than baseline states), if their scales contain mixtures of categories for existence and gradation, and if indexes of existence cover a variety of diagnostic phenomena. The management of these problems is discussed in the subsections that follow.

14.5.2.1. *Indexes of Outcome*

Status indexes can refer to certain outcomes occurring after an intervention. The outcome is a status if it is cited (in relative isolation) without regard to the patient's previous condition. For example, if we say that the patient had mild chest pain and a blood pressure of 140/90 after treatment, the outcome is reported as a status. If we say that pain has been reduced from severe to mild, and that blood pressure has fallen 20 mmHg, the outcome would be reported as a change. Outcomes that are expressed as changes—such as remissions, recrudescences, increases, or decreases—will be cited later under *indexes of change.*

14.5.2.2. *Scales for Existence and Gradation*

In describing existence or gradation or both, status indexes can be expressed in four types of scale that may sometimes be confusing when a scale of existence has gradations, or when a scale of gradation also includes existence. The scales are simple and easy to understand when existence is cited in direct binary fashion as **yes/no** or **present/absent,** and when gradation is cited in a direct list of magnitudes such as **mild, moderate, severe.** A scale of existence becomes more complex if the index refers to a relative certainty or probability of existence. The scale for such an index might contain ordinal grades of existence such as the categories **definitely present, probably present, uncertain whether present or absent, probably absent,** and **definitely absent.** A gradation scale becomes complex if the index refers to existence and gradation simultaneously, with the scale expressed as **none, mild, moderate, severe.** The null-based category allows the single scale to express existence if the entity is absent, and to grade magnitude if the entity is present. For purposes of classification, gradation indexes that contain a null-based category can be listed among the gradation group.

14.5.2.3. *Indexes of Existence*

The most common formal indexes of existence are used for diagnostic purposes. The indexes can appear as diagnostic criteria for specific diseases, as diagnostic marker tests, or in differential diagnosis. Indexes of existence are also often cited—without being called diagnostic criteria—for specific clinical disorders or symptoms that are not regarded as diseases.

Indexes of existence are well illustrated by the *diagnostic criteria* that have been developed for many diseases, such as rheumatic fever,[3] myocardial infarction,[92] or tuberculosis.[6] Although the output scale may be a simple binary expression of **yes/no,** diagnostic criteria indexes can have a highly complex structure in the way that the components are chosen and aggregated.

Although laboratory tests—such as carcinoembryonic antigen, alpha-fetoprotein, and serum calcium level—have been the prime focus of research, a *diagnostic marker* can be a clinimetric index of existence if it comes from clinical data, such as different forms of chest pain or certain combinations of symptoms and physical signs. Diagnostic markers are usually evaluated for the accuracy with which they act as surrogates in identifying the presence of a particular disease during screening or other medical activities. The results are usually expressed in such statistical calculations as *sensitivity* and *specificity*.[54]

Another type of index of existence is formed by clinical criteria (when available) or multivariate models (such as discriminant function analysis) that have been used to produce *indexes of differential diagnosis*. The input consists of information regarding a patient's clinical, demographic, and/or paraclinical status. The output is a score or category that assigns a patient to one of several diagnostic groups, or that indicates a probability for the likelihood of different diagnostic possibilities.

When a disorder such as "severe GI bleeding," or a symptom such as "headache" or "angina pectoris," is used to circumscribe admission to a particular study, the investigators will often list the diagnostic criteria that served as indexes of existence for these entities. In many other circumstances, however, the existence of various "non-disease" entities is cited in a binary global scale (such as **yes/no)** with no criteria offered to demarcate the decisions. Although nondescript, such indexes of existence sometimes warrant taxonomic attention.

Indexes referring to primary, secondary, or other manifestations of disease can be subclassified, if desired, according to the context in which they appear. For example, the *existence* of angina pectoris—cited as substernal chest pain provoked by exertion and relieved by rest—is almost always a primary manifestation of coronary disease. Most other clinical manifestations of coronary disease are secondary. They arise from disorders such as cardiac arrhythmias or congestive heart failure that can also be produced by ailments other than coronary disease.

An index that defines the existence of diarrhea would cite it as a primary manifestation in a study of gastroenteritis, diarrhea, or constipation, but as a secondary manifestation in a study of peptic ulcer. The subclassification of indexes of existence for disorders or symptoms will thus depend on the context in which the index is used.

14.5.3. PROBLEMS IN INDEXES OF CHANGE OR COMPARISON

Indexes of change contain single ratings that are used to compare a before and after state in a single person, or the pattern noted in a successive series of ratings, or sometimes a direct contrast of two people who usually have been matched for the comparison. Like indexes of status, indexes of change can refer to existence or gradation. A change in existence can be cited in such terms as **disappearance, remission, reappearance, recurrence, exacerbation,** or **relapse.** A change in gradation is cited with the comparative expressions contained in such terms as **better, rise, same, decrease of one grade, improved,** or **deteriorated.** Either the change itself, or the pattern noted in a series of ratings, can sometimes be described with ratings of desirability such as **excellent, good, fair, poor, normal,** or **abnormal.**

The subsections that follow refer to problems in classification that can arise for indexes referring to changes in existence, to patterns of change, and to changes in gradation.

14.5.3.1. *Changes in Existence*

Criteria for diagnosing the disappearance or reappearance of a particular ailment will often differ from the criteria used for its existence. In patients with cancer, a special index of change will be needed to denote what is meant by a *remission*. In patients who have already had an episode of acute rheumatic fever or acute myocardial infarction, a *recurrence* will require separate diagnostic criteria, often different from those with which the original occurrence was diagnosed. In patients with ailments such as peptic ulcer, rheumatoid arthritis, or asthma, a *relapse* or *exacerbation* will require criteria that indicate both the lowered level of previous "activity" for the ailment, as well as the level of rise that warrants the decision about a recrudescence.

14.5.3.2. *Indexes of Pattern*

A patient's response to a therapeutic intervention is often described with a single index that describes the pattern noted in a series of single-state ratings. The data may be obtained as repeated measurements of blood pressure, in pain scores recorded with a daily diary, in weekly examinations of joints, or with other methods of observation.

When the pattern of observations is summarized with a single index, the summary can be a total sum of the ratings, an average (or mean) value for the sum, a description of their trend (with a regression coefficient or in words such as **rising** or **stable),** or an appraisal of the pattern's desirability as **excellent, fair, poor,** etc. Other terms, such as **normal** or **abnormal,** might be used for the pattern of values seen in the series of measurements called a *glucose tolerance curve.*

Indexes of pattern are most often used to describe a patient's outcome after therapy, but they can sometimes be used for a baseline state before treatment. For example, the baseline value of a patient's pre-therapeutic blood pressure can be selected as the most recent value, an average of several preceding values, an average of the values that are most common or stable, or in some other method used to review the pattern and to arrive at a single value that will be regarded as the baseline. The pattern of manifestations for angina pectoris is often used to label its baseline state as **stable, unstable,** or **crescendo.**

14.5.3.3. *Changes in Gradation*

Changes in gradation can be derived from an analysis of repeated measurements of the same single-state index or with a separate *transition index,* devoted specifically to the change itself.

In the most common process, before and after ratings of status are directly compared. The result is usually cited as an increment (or decrement) such as **+10, rise of 10, −6, fall of 6, no change, increase of one grade,** or with other comparative terms. Sometimes the change is expressed as the trend in a pattern of several repeated ratings, such as **rapid rise** or **gradual fall.**

In other circumstances, however, the change is cited in a separate monadic transition index, which is devoted exclusively to rating the change itself without using specific dyadic components (such as before or after values), or polyadic components of single-state ratings on multiple occasions. In a monadic transition, the change is rated in a comparative category, such as **better, same, worse, greatly improved, slightly deteriorated,** or with an appropriate visual analog scale whose linear extremes might be **much worse** and **completely improved**—but no specific attention is given to any single-state ratings for the current condition or the previous conditions. Those conditions are obviously considered by the person who rates the transition, but the individual single-state ratings are not specifically identified.

Monadic transition indexes are a form of measurement that is probably unique in clinimetrics. They do not occur (because they are not needed) in traditional forms of laboratory measurement that provide dimensional expressions for single variables. The transition indexes become desirable for the many clinimetric phenomena that are cited in categorical scales or in scales that contain a composite mixture of many variables. The main advantages of transition indexes, as discussed earlier in Section 5.2.4.2, is the ability to detect changes that may be missed if the scale of a single-state index is too coarse or if the discrimination of change is obscured by the many components and aggregations of a composite multivariate index.

14.5.4. INDEXES OF PREDICTION

In the strictest form of construction, indexes of prediction have three parts: a status index that describes the baseline state for which the prediction is being made; an outcome index that describes the subsequent state or change whose likelihood is being predicted; and an expression that denotes the relationship between the two. An example of the three parts is shown in the statement: **"survival rate at one year** (the outcome event) is **30%** (the relationship) for **patients with Stage III cancer** (the baseline state)." In the actual classification of these parts, **Stage III** is the category of the predictive index, **30% chance** is the prediction itself, and **survival at one year** is the outcome that is being predicted.

Not all predictive indexes are expressed in so complete a manner, however. In many statements of prognosis, clinicians may use terms such as **good, poor,** or **hopeless,** without specifying the predicted outcome, although the outcome is evident in predictions such as **moribund,** or **impending myocardial infarction.**

In formal studies of predictive indexes, however, the three constituent parts are usually specified, but different formats may be used for the specifications. Sometimes the outcome is cited as a variable rather than an event, and the predictive relationship is expressed as a correlation coefficient between the baseline index and the outcome variable. Thus, survival might be cited as correlating well with age. If the prediction emerges from a multivariate mathematical model, the predictive index includes several variables, each of which may have a univariate or multivariate role. For the univariate role, the relationship to the outcome is expressed for that variable alone. For the multivariate role, the relationship to the outcome is expressed for the effect of that variable in simultaneous combination with the other predictor variables.

For purposes of classification within a particular ailment or condition, predictive indexes are best cited according to the particular outcome that is being predicted. The individual predictor variables can then be cited according to their univariate and multivariate roles.

14.5.5. GUIDELINE INDEXES

Guideline indexes can be classified according to the particular action (in therapy, choice of diagnostic tests, etc.) for which they offer directions. Further citations can be used to indicate whether the directions are based on clinical judgment alone, or to classify any documentary evidence offered for the value or validity of the directions in the guideline.

Chapter 15

Summary and Conclusions

For readers who like to have a synopsis of what they have read, this chapter contains a summary of the preceding fourteen chapters, together with some additional conclusions.

Nomenclature and Functional Classification

Clinimetric indexes are arbitrary ratings for the diverse phenomena of clinical care that are observed subjectively and that cannot be expressed in dimensional numbers. The indexes have diverse roles in clinical medicine. Indexes of status contain diagnostic criteria for existence, or graded ratings for relative magnitude or severity of symptoms, diseases, functional capacity, and other clinical conditions. Indexes of change describe alterations that are determined from successive ratings of a condition's status, or from special transition scales aimed at describing change itself. Indexes of prediction are used for prognostic estimations; and guideline indexes, which are sometimes called "protocols" or "algorithms," offer instructions for decisions that lead to diagnostic and therapeutic actions. The data produced by clinimetric indexes are used for diverse activities in observing, planning, evaluating, and statistically analyzing the results of patient care.

The indexes are important because they describe human sensations, reactions, and judgments that are often regarded as too "soft" to be included in statistical or other "scientific" analyses of patient care. The omission of the soft clinical information is detrimental for both humanism and science in modern medicine. Humanistically, the focus on "hard" data does not include suitable attention to distress, relief, comfort, gratification, and other distinctively human desires and goals. Scientifically, in the absence of suitable soft data, the patients who are the observed "material" are not identified reproducibly or effectively. The identifications are inadequate because some of the most cogent distinctions in diagnosis, prognosis, and therapy depend on patterns of symptoms, severity of illness, effects of co-morbidity, functional abilities, and other clinical phenomena that must be described with soft data, and that will not be accounted for in the hard information.

A common reason why soft clinical information is often scientifically disdained is that the information comes from subjective observations and is expressed without the formal standards applied for measuring hard data in laboratory work. The problem of subjective observation is actually less of a scientific obstacle than the lack of standardized expression because other forms of subjectively observed data—obtained via histopathology, radiology, and electron microscopy—have received widespread scientific acceptance. The standardization problem, which has been a prime topic in this book, can be resolved if a formal process is established for the development of clinimetric indexes. The process will have to differ substantially, however, from what is used in other forms of measurement because the indexes have so many different structures, purposes, and functions.

Principles of Structure

Clinimetric indexes are constructed from component variables that are often expressed in nominal, binary, ordinal, or quasi-dimensional rating scales that differ from dimensional measurements. In some instances, the original scale of a component variable is transformed into a different scale before the component enters the index. A single index often contains many component variables, which are sometimes organized into axes (or "subscales") before being arranged into the output scale of the index.

The output scale formed by a combination of component variables can be cited as a tandem profile or as an aggregation. In a tandem profile, a separate rating appears for each component axis. In an aggregation, the component ratings are joined into a single set of output categories that form a new scale. The aggregations can be arranged as additive scores or Boolean clusters, and the arrangements can be organized as summations or in a ranked hierarchical format.

The diverse scales of expression, multiple component variables, and composite patterns of aggregation create major complexities in construction and evaluation. The strategies used to deal with these complexities will differ substantially from the simpler methods that can be applied when conventional laboratory measurements are cited in standard dimensional scales for single variables. In a composite clinimetric index, such attributes as the scope, discrimination, coherence, and stipulated aggregation of the output scale are crucial features that seldom need consideration in conventional laboratory measurements.

Choice of Component Variables

Because of the need to consider the specific clinical purpose and setting for which each index is intended, the component variables for clinimetric indexes are chosen in a manner that differs from other forms of measurement. In laboratory work, each measurement is expressed in the same way no matter how the data may be used, but clinimetric indexes may require different components for different usages. In psychosocial measurements, the components that enter each index are often selected after a long list of candidate "items" has been evaluated and tested. In clinimetric indexes, however, the component variables are often chosen directly from a review of past clinical experience, followed by a "dissection" of the "intuition" with which the pertinent phenomena were appraised. The process is eased by the fact that each phenomenon or "construct" being described in clinical work has usually become well recognized and established *before* attempts are made to express it with an index. After being selected, the component variables are further refined to include the appropriate forms of intrinsic or extrinsic evidence and to aim at an appropriate focus for the interpersonal exchange.

When many candidates are considered as possible component variables for a new index, the most important ones are often selected mainly by ordinary clinical judgment, but "importance" can also be determined with various mathematical models or with combinations of clinico-statistical judgment.

Organization of Output Scale

When the component variables are combined to form an output scale, the scale should contain an exhaustive scope of mutually exclusive categories, a suitable location for all the component parts and combinations, and realistic values. The output scale will be defective if it produces excessive, inadequate, or obscure discrimination, or if it does not offer an effective method of discerning changes in state. Some of these problems can be avoided if the index focuses on a smaller number of crucial components or is constructed as a separate transition index, intended specifically to identify changes.

Biometric coherence, another valuable feature of a multi-component index, is achieved if the attributes combined in the composite categories have a plausible biologic meaning and also have similar statistical properties. Another desirable attribute is "transparency," which allows the distinctive contents of the composite categories to be easily discerned from the output expression. Transparency is impaired if too many variables are combined in a single citation.

The three attributes of biologic plausibility, statistical isometry, and scientific transparency are all desirable, but they often involve conflicts that keep all three from being attainable in a single index. Consequently, the investigator will often have to choose which of the competing goals should be given priority. The problems that arise during these choices will re-appear in the subsequent discussion of conflicts in statistical, psychosocial, and clinical goals for clinimetric indexes.

Role of Patients' Collaboration

Regardless of how the component variables are chosen and combined, the results of many indexes are often unsatisfactory because an important feature has been neglected: the collaboration of the patient. To give accurate or appropriate responses either to an interviewer or to a self-administered questionnaire, the patient must be sufficiently cooperative, alert, and comprehending. In some important instances, however, the responses are accepted without suitable evaluation of the patient's mental condition.

If the index requires performance of a physical task—such as climbing stairs, breathing in a special way, or working at a particular job—the magnitude of the task should be clearly specified and the task should be clearly understood by the patient. If the task is not accomplished, the reasons for non-accomplishment should be differentiated into clinical, phobic, economic, or other reasons; and a distinction should be made between threshold levels or maximum tolerance levels for magnitude of performance. Since the magnitude of a performed task can usually be raised if effort is decreased or if social support is increased, an assessment of magnitude alone will be inadequate if effort and other sources of support are not suitably considered. For example, angina pectoris can easily be "cured" if the patient works much more slowly at the same task that formerly evoked the angina when done rapidly.

Another important aspect of collaboration is the patient's choice of a preferred focus when multiple manifestations or disabilities are the target of therapy. The patient's selection of such a focus can help orient a suitable direction for both the treatment itself and the index with which the treatment is evaluated.

Global Indexes and Scales

A unique feature that differentiates clinimetric from laboratory measurements is the frequent use of global indexes and scales. These indexes are expressed in visual analog, ordinal, binary, or nominal categories, but operational criteria are not provided to demarcate the choice of each category. The indexes are most commonly used for broad "global" ratings of complex phenomena such as severity of illness, post-therapeutic improvement, or health status, but can also be applied for more specific clinical entities such as severity of dyspnea, severity of pain, or degree of cardiac enlargement.

The main advantage of the global indexes is their simplicity and their direct focus on the selected phenomenon; their main disadvantage is the absence of the stipulations needed for scientific reproducibility. The latter disadvantage is often reduced if the same person repeatedly uses the same index, if the global index describes transitions rather than single states, if certain precautions (such as "blinding") are used to enhance objectivity, or if comprehension of categorical ratings is aided by graphic displays.

Because of convenience and ease, global indexes are constantly used in clinical communication, but they are often shunned in scientific analyses because the data are regarded as soft and unreliable. The hard data that are used instead, however, may have high scientific quality but may not offer suitable descriptions of the selected phenomena. The achievement of both sensibility and standardization in the same index is often difficult, and the desire of attaining both goals may lead to major unrecognized conflicts when mathematical, psychometric, and clinical strategies are used in constructing and evaluating clinimetric indexes. The collaborators from the different disciplines may not realize that they have different goals, and may not perceive the need to specify priorities or make suitable compromises when the disparate goals are pursued.

Goals of Statistical Methods

Statistical strategies can be used in at least two different ways in the construction of clinimetric indexes. In one approach, if the index is formulated by judgmental combination, statistical procedures can review a collection of existing data and can identify (or confirm) the variables that seem most important for inclusion as components of the index. In a second approach, the index itself is constructed from the data by a statistical technique that chooses the important variables, assigns weights to their coefficients, and combines them into a score or cluster.

With either approach, the strategies depend on mathematical models that summarize the data in a selected (usually "linear") pattern and that evaluate the variables according to their apparent effect in reducing statistical variance. Although the results may indicate the "important" variables, the importance depends on basic judgments that are mathematical rather than clinical or scientific. The judgments involve arbitrary decisions in choosing a mathematical model, reacting to violations of basic assumptions that underlie the model, selecting variables to be explored for "interactions," establishing guidelines for the computer operations, identifying elemental variables and "unions" of variables, designating systems to code the data, and interpreting the results. Because the results are usually displayed as coefficients of association and expressions for reduction in variance, the investigator may not see direct tabulations for the actual impact of the individual variables or combinations of variables.

The statistical procedures have been highly successful in circumstances where only a few variables are being analyzed. When many variables are under consideration, the results have the advantage of coming from a standardized mathematical procedure. The disadvantage is that the procedure makes all its decisions with a mathematical orientation. The orientation does not consider biologic plausibility or clinical connotations; it is often strongly affected by the amount (rather than scientific content) of the data; and it is often difficult for clinicians to understand and apply.

Goals of Psychosocial Methods

The psychosocial strategies for constructing indexes are often aimed at specific scientific goals, such as achieving a unidimensional variable, with a consistently monotonic pattern, and equal intervals between categories on the output scale. Although desirable for developing indexes about personal attitudes and beliefs, these goals may differ sharply from what is desired in a clinimetric index. The clinician may deliberately want to combine multiple different variables, knowing that the result will not form a consistently monotonic pattern, and seeking an ordinal set of graded ratings that will not have equal intervals between categories. In addition, when psychosocial methods are used to develop a hierarchical ("Gutmann scale") arrangement, the mathematical formulations may differ substantially from the judgmental approaches with which a clinician might organize the rankings.

In certain psychosocial approaches, personal opinions may be solicited with indirect or general questions such as "Do you like doctors?" rather than with direct, targeted questions such as "Do you like *your* doctor?" The indirect strategy may be desirable for certain types of interrogation, but the answer may not always reflect the particular opinions that were sought.

Perhaps the main advantage of the psychosocial approach is that it is accompanied by an established background of "theory" to justify the methods and goals. Lacking an articulated set of principles and "theory" for their own aims in constructing indexes, clinicians may not recognize the occasional or frequent disparities between psychosocial and clinical goals, and may not provide a suitable orientation for the psychosocial-clinical collaboration.

Theory and Evaluation of Sensibility

A theory can be developed for the goal of sensibility in clinimetric indexes by considering five main features of each index: its purpose and framework, overt format, face validity, content validity, and ease of usage.

The purpose and framework are evaluated to check that the index is suitable for its desired function (in describing status, change, etc.); that its novel features or improvements are justified; and that it is applicable for the clinical setting in which its use is planned.

The overt format of the index should be comprehensible, with a relatively small number of coherent variables; the results should be replicable via operating instructions that are clear and carried out in an unbiased manner; and the output scale should be suitably comprehensive in its scope of categories and suitably discriminating among the categories.

The "face validity" of the index requires an appropriate direct focus for the interpersonal exchange, a suitable emphasis in the choice of basic evidence, components that are biologically coherent, and proper attention to the role of the patient's personal collaboration. The "content validity" of the index is determined by checking that it has not omitted important variables or included unimportant ones; that the component variables have been given suitable weights; that the elemental scales are satisfactory for each variable; and that the basic data have good quality.

The ease of usage depends on the time, effort, potential hazards, and type of personnel needed to employ the index.

The various features just cited can be arranged into a list of 21 principles that can be used, somewhat like a "review of systems" in a patient's clinical examination, as a background strategy or theory for the evaluation of sensibility in clinimetric indexes.

Evaluation of Consistency

An essential feature of quality in scientific data is the achievement of similar results when the same measurement is repeated by the same or another observer. Because the similar results may all be wrong, the term *reliability* is not a good name for this attribute of the data. The word *consistency* seems preferable to *repeatability* or *reproducibility,* particularly at times when the exact circumstances in which the measurement is made can be neither repeated nor reproduced.

Consistency of a measurement process has paramount scientific importance because inconsistent results will seldom warrant further appraisal. The consistency of the process is usually checked externally for observer variability within or among the users, but composite indexes can also be checked for internal consistency in the inter-relationship among component variables. The different components can be checked for "split-half reliability" or for the generalized inter-correlations calculated with statistical procedures such as Cronbach's alpha.

The most customary and conventional assessments of consistency are devoted to observer variability. Before any formal tests begin, efforts can be made to reduce observer variability by developing clear instructions for use of the index, and by improving the operational instructions after exploration of the disagreements noted in pilot studies. The disagreements can arise from variability in the input, the procedure, or the users. The operating instructions must provide both ingredient criteria for the basic observations and conversion criteria for their transformation into the available ratings.

When tested in formal field trials, observer variability can be noted with several statistical expressions. They can cite the average magnitudes of disagreement, or the percentages of absolute agreement or weighted disagreement. An alternative approach, which contains a correction for agreement that might occur by chance in categorical data, is to cite the concordance associations by calculating kappa or weighted kappa. In all of these statistical expressions, arbitrary numerical boundaries must be established to delineate gradations of good or poor agreement.

Field trials of observer variability have often been omitted when an index seemed to perform well first in pilot studies and later in practical applications. The trials are particularly desirable if substantial acts of subjective judgment are involved in the basic observations or their subsequent conversions.

Evaluation of Validity

Because a "gold standard" measurement seldom exists to offer a definitive result, the accuracy of clinimetric indexes can seldom be evaluated. The appraisal is usually devoted to validity, which is examined in two different ways. In one approach, called "criterion validity," the new index is checked against a gold standard if it is available; otherwise some other indexes, which are well accepted as measurements of the same or an analogous phenomenon, are used as the substitute criterion.

In a second type of appraisal, called "construct validity," the index is checked for its suitability in describing the concept (or "construct") of the selected phenomenon. These phenomena can range from clinical ideas about congestive heart failure, to general classifications of health status, and to psychometric beliefs about intelligence. Construct validity can be appraised in at least three ways. In the first method, the purpose of the analysis is to help demonstrate the existence of a construct created by mathematical procedures such as factor analysis. In the second method, which is sometimes called "discriminant validity," the goal is to show that the new index does something different from existing indexes, by demonstrating its dissociation (rather than correlation) with those indexes. In the third method, which is particularly common for clinimetric indexes, the index receives a "validation by application." In this procedure, the index is evaluated according to its actual performance in an appropriate research study. For example, an index for rating pain would be validated by application if its results suitably differentiate a known effective analgesic agent from a placebo in a clinical trial of pain relief.

The statistical expressions for validity often employ measurements of association, but additional tactics (such as the calculation of sensitivity, specificity, and likelihood ratios) may be used if the index is being checked for accuracy in diagnostic identifications or prognostic predictions. Two important policy decisions for these evaluations involve the management of uncertain results and the choices of boundaries to demarcate abnormality, success, or other categorical zones.

Design and Evaluation of Field Trials

Although field trials are needed to produce the data that are statistically evaluated for consistency and validity, the trials themselves seldom receive the intensive attention given to the statistical results. Nevertheless, because the trials are designed to test a group of people for a particular purpose, the structure of the trials is crucially important for deciding whether the statistical results are pertinent and generalizable.

In a study of consistency, the choice of the observed group, the participating observers, and the methods of comparison must be unbiased, suitable for the main objective, and applicable to the subsequent groups to which the results would pertain. In a study of validity, the assembled evidence should also be aimed at the kinds of patients and clinical settings in which the index would subsequently be applied.

Field trials are also used for a type of validation that serves to confirm the original studies of "validity." The index is often developed from a previous set of data called the *training, developmental,* or *generating* set. The results are then checked and confirmed in a different group of people, who are called the *challenge* or *test* set. Because this type of confirmation is often essential but often omitted, many indexes have been validated within their generating set, but have not received the additional cogent validation that would come from a challenge set.

Regardless of whether the field trial is concerned with consistency or validity (or both), the input to the trial should contain a suitably broad and representative spectrum of patients, who may need further analysis in appropriate subgroups. The indexes being compared should receive a similar input, avoiding problems that may arise from unstable phenomena, sequential-ordering bias, or changes in clinical setting. The contrasted operating procedures should each be carried out properly and compared in an unbiased manner.

Inadequately structured field trials are accompanied by three main hazards. A false negative conclusion, in which a potentially useful index is dismissed as valueless, can arise if the field trial is done prematurely, before the index has been improved in pilot studies, or if the trial contains unsuitable groups or biased comparisons. A false positive conclusion, which claims value for a relatively useless index, is particularly likely to occur if the comparative observational processes were biased, but can also occur when large sample sizes produce "statistical significance" for relatively unimpressive quantitative distinctions. Perhaps the most common hazard, however, is the over-interpretation of high statistical results for "reliability" and "validity." Investigators seeking an index for a new research project may check the field-trial statistics, be impressed with them, use the index in the new study, and only then discover that the index had not been checked for its sensibility. The index may have been insensitive to change, aimed at the wrong focus, intended for patients in different clinical settings, or otherwise inadequate for its assigned role.

These problems can be avoided if investigators recognize that statistical coefficients of reliability and validity should not be accepted without evaluation of the field trial from which they emanated. In some instances, the investigators may be better off in making the effort to construct a new index, rather than using a "validated" index that works improperly.

Taxonomy of Clinimetric Indexes

For comparative evaluations and classifications, clinimetric indexes can be divided into two main groups: the *ailment-oriented* and the *general*. General indexes refer to general health and functional states that are not distinctive for a particular clinical disease or condition. Ailment-oriented indexes refer to specific diseases, conditions, or other clinical manifestations that are the conventional phenomena observed in patient care. The indexes can be ailment-specific (producing diagnostic criteria for a particular disease or descriptions of symptoms distinctive to that disease), or disorder-specific (describing clinical manifestations that are not unique to a single disease). Ailment-oriented indexes can also describe systemic symptoms (such as anorexia and weight loss), the temporal attributes of clinical manifestations, the co-morbidity of associated diseases, or such ancillary features as additional therapy.

Since all of the ailment-oriented indexes can be used to describe patients in the different parts of the spectrum of an ailment, the term *spectral index* can be applied for combinations that contain several different types of ailment-oriented indexes. The term *hybrid index* can be used when an ailment-oriented index is combined with a general index or with paraclinical data from laboratory tests, radiography, or other technologic procedures.

Additional taxonomic issues involve classification for the format of uncalibrated or global scales that can be applied for many different topics, for the management of demarcated indexes produced as aggregates of global scales, and other variations in conventional structure.

Conclusions

For new technology to be applied with human values and goals, the data under analysis cannot be confined to information obtained exclusively with technologic procedures. The data must include accounts of clinical phenomena that reflect the human values and goals. Among such phenomena are the symptoms and other overt manifestations of disease, the associated disabilities and other functional impairments, and various reactions by patients, families, and physicians to these phenomena. This soft information can be noted and hardened if suitable clinimetric indexes are developed for the activities.

The strategies and structures of clinimetric rating scales can readily be improved, although the procedures will be different from those used to improve scientific quality in conventional laboratory methods of measurement. During the clinimetric activities in construction and evaluation of indexes, conflicts may sometimes arise between two competing goals. One of these goals is to achieve a sensibility that makes the index easy to use and well suited for its distinctive purpose. The other goal is to have a standardization that makes the index produce consistent, validated results.

Although standardization and sensibility are both desirable goals, they may not always be readily achieved in the same index. The ease of usage desired for clinical sensibility may not be compatible with the extensive details often required for standardization. When the relatively few components of a sensible index are chosen according to clinical judgment, the choice may not have the standardization provided by a mathematical analysis of multiple candidate variables. When the face validity and content validity of a clinimetric index are qualitatively appraised for sensibility, the result will lack the quantitative prestige provided by standard statistical formulas for measuring criterion validity and construct validity. The direct, on-target simplicity of a global scale for describing a complex phenomenon may be sensible but unstandardized, whereas a reliable, validated composite combination of demarcated ratings for multiple component variables may be standardized but not sensible.

The potential conflict between the goals of sensibility and standardization will therefore often require decisions in setting priorities. Certain strategies of statistics and psychosocial science can offer valuable guidance in the quest for standardization, but the clinician's knowledge of purpose, setting, and content is invaluable for achieving sensibility and for giving it priority when crucial decisions are made. The likelihood of achieving both goals will be increased if the clinical investigators and their collaborating consultants become thoughtfully familiar with both sets of goals, with the methods of approaching them, and with the need for both flexibility and ingenuity in the approaches.

Like clinical practice itself, the development of clinimetric indexes requires an intricate combination of artful humanism and rigorous science. The attainment of that combination can help restore, preserve, and augment the role of personal and clinical phenomena as the center of attention when technologic clinical science is used in humanistic patient care.

References

1. Adami HO, Björklund O, Enander LK, Gustavsson S, Lööf L, Nordahl A, Rosén A. Cimetidine or propantheline combined with antacid therapy for short-term treatment of duodenal ulcer. Dig Dis Sci 1982;27:388-93.
2. Aitken RCB. Measurement of feelings using visual analogue scales. Proc Roy Soc Med 1969;62:989-93.
3. American Heart Association Committee on Rheumatic Fever and Bacterial Endocarditis. Jones criteria (revised) for guidance in the diagnosis of rheumatic fever. Circulation 1984;69:203A-8A.
4. American Joint Committee for Cancer Staging and End Results Reporting. Manual for staging of cancer. Chicago, 1977.
5. Apgar V. A proposal for a new method of evaluation of the newborn infant. Anesth Analg 1953;32:260-7.
6. Bates JH. Diagnosis of tuberculosis. Chest (suppl) 1979;76:757-63.
7. Bennett AE, Ritchie K. Questionnaires in medicine. New York: Oxford Univ Press, 1975.
8. Bergner M, Bobbitt RA, Carter WB, Gilson BS. The Sickness Impact Profile: Development and final revision of a health status measure. Med Care 1981;19: 787-805.
9. Bernard C. An introduction to the study of experimental medicine, translated by Greene HC, published in paperback. New York: Collier Books, 1961. (Originally published in 1865)
10. Bishop YMM, Fienberg SE, Holland PW. Discrete multivariate analysis: Theory and practice. Cambridge: MIT Press, 1975.
11. Bock RD, Jones LV. The measurement and prediction of judgment and choice. San Francisco: Holden-Day, 1968.
12. Boring EG. The beginning and growth of measurement in psychology. In: Woolf H, ed. Quantification. A history of the meaning of measurement in the natural and social sciences. New York: The Bobbs-Merrill Co, Inc. 1961:108-27.

257

13. Charlson ME, Feinstein AR. The auxometric dimension. A new method for using rate growth in prognostic staging of breast cancer. JAMA 1974;228:180-5.
14. Cicchetti DV, Showalter D, Tyrer PJ. The effect of number of rating scale categories on levels of interrater reliability: A Monte Carol investigation. Appl Psych Measurement 1985;9:31-6.
15. Clarke PRF, Spear FG. Reliability and sensitivity in the self-assessment of well-being. Bull Brit Psychol Soc 1964;17:18A.
16. College of American Pathologists Committee on Nomenclature and Classification of Disease. Systematized nomenclature of pathology. Chicago: College of American Pathologists, 1965.
17. Comstock GW, Tockman MS, Helsing KJ, Hennesy KM. Standardized respiratory questionnaires: Comparison of the old with the new. Am Rev Respir Dis 1979;119:45-53.
18. Conn HO, Smith HW, Brodoff M. Observer variation in the endoscopic diagnosis of esophageal varices: A prospective investigation of the diagnostic validity of esophagoscopy. N Engl J Med 1965;272:830-4.
19. Cooney LM, Wells CK, Miller RL, Feinstein AR. An improved index for predicting patients' needs for assistance in chronic care. Clin Res 1984;32:477A.
20. Council on Clinical Classifications. International classification of diseases, 9th revision, Clinical modification. Ann Arbor: Commission on Professional and Hospital Activities, 1980.
21. Council on the Kidney in Cardiovascular Disease, American Heart Association. Criteria for the evaluation of the severity of established renal disease. Ann Intern Med 1971;75:251-2.
22. Craig CF, Nichols HJ. The effect of the ingestion of alcohol on the result of the complement fixation test in syphilis. JAMA 1911;57:474-6.
23. Craig CF. The practical application of the Wasserman test in the diagnosis and control of treatment of syphilis. Am J Syphilis 1917;1:192-210.
24. Criteria Committee of the New York Heart Association, Inc. Diseases of the heart and blood vessels: Nomenclature and criteria for diagnosis, 6th ed. Boston: Little, Brown, 1964.
25. Cronbach LJ. Coefficient alpha and the internal structure of tests. Psychometrika 1951;16:297-334.
26. Dawes RM. Fundamentals of attitude measurement. New York: John Wiley and Sons, 1972.
27. Detre KM, Wright E, Murphy ML, Takaro T. Observer agreement in evaluating coronary angiograms. Circulation 1975;52:979-86.
28. Detsky AS, Johnston N, McLaughlin JR, Drucker DJ, Sasson Z, Scott JG, Forbath N, Hilliard JR. A multifactorial cardiac risk index for patients undergoing noncardiac surgery. Clin Res 1985;33:247A.
29. Deyo RA. Measuring functional outcomes in therapeutic trials for chronic disease. Controlled Clin Trials 1984;5:223-40.
30. Dillman DA. Mail and telephone surveys. The total design method. New York: John Wiley and Sons, 1978.
31. Dorn HF, Moriyama IM. Uses and significance of multiple cause tabulations for mortality statistics. Am J Public Health 1964;54:400-6.

32. Downie WW, Leatham PA, Rhind VM, Wright V, Branco JA, Anderson JA. Studies with pain rating scales. Ann Rheum Dis 1978;37:378–81.

33. Duthie JJR, Brown PE, Knox JDE, Thompson M. Course and prognosis in rheumatoid arthritis. Ann Rheum Dis 1957;16:411–22.

34. Ehrenberg ASC. Data reduction. New York: John Wiley and Sons, 1975.

35. Eysenck HJ, Crown S. An experimental study in opinion-attitude methodology. Int J Opinion Attitude Res 1949;3:47–86.

36. Feigenbaum SL, Masi AT, Kaplan SB. Prognosis in rheumatoid arthritis. A longitudinal study of newly diagnosed younger adult patients. Am J. Med 1979;66:377–84.

37. Feinstein AR, Wood HF, Spagnuolo M, Taranta A, Jonas S, Kleinberg E, Tursky E. Rheumatic fever in children and adolescents: A long-term epidemiologic study of subsequent prophylaxis, streptococcal infections, and clinical sequelae. VII. Cardiac changes and sequelae. Ann Intern Med 1964;(suppl 5)60:87–123.

38. Feinstein AR. Clinical judgment. Baltimore: Williams and Wilkins, 1967. (Reprinted copy available from Robert E. Krieger Co., Melbourne, Florida.)

39. Feinstein AR, Stern E. Clinical effects of recurrent attacks of acute rheumatic fever: A prospective epidemiologic study of 105 episodes. J Chron Dis 1967;20:13–27.

40. Feinstein AR. Taxonorics. I. Formulation of criteria; II. Formats and coding systems for data processing. Arch Intern Med 1970;126:679–93,1053–67.

41. Feinstein AR. The pre-therapeutic classification of co-morbidity in chronic disease. J Chron Dis 1970;23:455–69.

42. Feinstein AR, Gelfman NA, Yesner R, with the collaboration of Auerbach O, Hackel DB, Pratt PC. Observer variability in histopathologic diagnosis of lung cancer. Am Rev Resp Dis 1970;101:671–84.

43. Feinstein AR. Clinical biostatistics: XII. On exorcising the ghost of Gauss and the curse of Kelvin. Clin Pharmacol Ther 1971;12:1003–16.

44. Feinstein AR. An analysis of diagnostic reasoning: I. The domains and disorders of clinical macrobiology; II. The strategy of intermediate decisions; III. The construction of clinical algorithms. Yale J Biol Med 1973;46:212–32,264–83; 1974;47:5–32.

45. Feinstein AR, Schimpff CR, Hull EW (with the technical assistance of HL Bidwell). A reappraisal of staging and therapy for patients with cancer of the rectum. I. Development of two systems of staging. Arch Intern Med 1975;135: 1441–53.

46. Feinstein AR. Clinical biostatistics: XXXVI. The persistent biometric problems of the UGDP study. Clin Pharmacol Ther 1976;19:472–85.

47. Feinstein AR. Clinical biostatistics. St. Louis: CV Mosby Co, 1977, chapters 26–29.

48. Feinstein AR, Schimpff CR, Andrews JF Jr, Wells CK. Cancer of the larynx: A new staging system and a re-appraisal of prognosis and treatment. J Chron Dis 1977;30:277–305.

49. Feinstein AR, Wells CK. A new clinical taxonomy for rating change in functional activities of patients with angina pectoris. Am Heart J 1977;93: 172–82.

50. Feinstein AR, Wells CK. Lung cancer staging: A critical evaluation. Clin Chest Med 1982;3:291–305.
51. Feinstein AR. The Jones criteria and the challenges of clinimetrics. Circulation 1982;66:1–5.
52. Feinstein AR. An additional basic science for clinical medicine: III. The challenges of comparison and measurement. Ann Intern Med 1983;99:705–12.
53. Feinstein AR. An additional basic science for clinical medicine: IV. The development of clinimetrics. Ann Intern Med 1983;99:843–8.
54. Feinstein AR. Clinical epidemiology. The architecture of clinical research. Philadelphia: WB Saunders, 1985.
55. Feinstein AR. Stochastic contrasts. In: Clinical epidemiology. Philadelphia: WB Saunders, 1985, chapter 9.
56. Feinstein AR. Diagnostic and spectral markers. In: Clinical epidemiology. Philadelphia: WB Saunders, 1985, chapter 25.
57. Feinstein AR. Editorial. Tempest in a P-pot? Hypertension 1985;7:313–8.
58. Feinstein AR, Sosin DM, Wells CK. The Will Rogers phenomenon: Stage migration and new diagnostic technology as a source of misleading statistics for survival in cancer. N Engl J Med 1985;312:1604–8.
59. Feinstein AR. Editorial. On classifying cancers while treating patients. Arch Intern Med 1985;145:1789–91.
60. Feinstein AR, Wells CK, Joyce CM, Josephy BR. The evaluation of sensibility and the role of patient collaboration in clinimetric indexes. Trans Assoc Am Physicians 1985;98:146–9.
61. Feinstein AR, Josephy BR, Wells CK. Scientific and clinical problems in indexes of functional disability. Ann Intern Med (In Press).
62. Feinstein AR. Indexes of congestive heart failure (in preparation).
63. Feinstein AR. Indexes of locomotor disease (in preparation).
64. Fink A, Kosecoff J, Chassin M, Brook RH. Consensus methods: Characteristics and guidelines for use. Am J Public Heath 1984;74:979–83.
65. Fleiss JL. Statistical methods for rates and proportions. New York: John Wiley and Sons, 1981.
66. Forrest WH Jr, Bellville JW, Seed JC, Houde RW, Wallenstein SL, Sunshine A, Laska E. A uniform method for collecting and processing analgesic data. Psychopharmacol Service Ctr Bull 1963;2:1–10.
67. Freyd M. The graphic rating scale. J Educ Psychol 1923;14:83–102.
68. Friedman M, Rosenman RH. Association of specific overt behavior pattern with blood and cardiovascular findings. JAMA 1959;169:1286–96.
69. Goldman L, Caldera DL, Nussbaum SR, Southwick FS, Krogstad D, Murray B, Burke DS, O'Malley TA, Goroll AH, Caplan CH, Nolan J, Carabello B, Slater EE. Multifactorial index of cardiac risk in noncardiac surgical procedures. N Engl J Med 1977;297:845–50.
70. Gould SG. The mismeasure of man. New York: WW Norton, 1981.
71. Granger CV, Gresham GE, eds. Functional assessment in rehabilitative medicine. Baltimore/London: Williams and Wilkins, 1984.
72. Greenfield S, Cretin S, Worthman LG, Dorey FJ, Solomon NE, Goldberg GA. Comparison of a criteria map to a criteria list in quality-of-care assessment for

patients with chest pain: The relation of each to outcome. Med Care 1981;19: 255–72.

73. Greenfield S, Kaplan S, Ware JE Jr. Expanding patient involvement in care. Effects on patient outcomes. Ann Intern Med 1985;102:520–8.

74. Greenspan RH, Ravin CE, Polansky SM, McLoud TC. Accuracy of the chest radiograph in diagnosis of pulmonary embolism. Invest Radiol 1982;17:539–43.

75. Guthrie HA, Guthrie GM. Factor analysis of nutritional status data from ten state nutrition surveys. Am J Clin Nutr 1976;29:1238–41.

76. Guttman L. A basis for scaling quantitative data. Am Sociol Rev 1944;9:139–50.

77. Guyatt GH, Pugsley SO, Sullivan MJ, Thompson PJ, Berman LB, Jones NL, Fallen EL, Taylor DW. Effect of encouragement on walking test performance. Thorax 1984;39:818–22.

78. Guyatt GH, Berman LB, Townsend M, Taylor DW. Should study subjects see their previous responses? J Chron Dis 1985;38:1003–7.

79. Hall J, Iannos J. Doubts about linear analogue scales. Br Med J 1984;289:498–9.

80. Hamilton M. Development of a rating scale for primary depressive illness. Br J Soc Clin Psychol 1967;6:278–96.

81. Hartigan J. Clustering algorithms. New York: John Wiley and Sons, 1975.

82. Hayes MHS, Patterson DG. Experimental development of the graphic rating method. Psychol Bull 1921;18:98–9.

83. Hewer AJH, Keele CA, Keele KD, Nathan PW. A clinical method of assessing analgesics. Lancet 1949;1:431–5.

84. Houde RW, Wallenstein SL, Rogers A. Clinical pharmacology of analgesics. 1. A method of assaying analgesic effect. Clin Pharmacol Ther 1960;1:163–74.

85. Houde RW. (Personal Communication)

86. Hulka BS, Zyzanski SJ, Cassel JC, Thompson SJ. Scale for the measurement of attitudes toward physicians and primary medical care. Med Care 1970;8:429–35.

87. Hulka BS, Kupper LL, Daly MB, Cassel JC, Schoen F. Correlates of satisfaction and dissatisfaction with medical care: A community perspective. Med Care 1975;13:648–58.

88. Huskisson EC, Shenfield GM, Taylor RT, Hart FD. A new look at ibuprofen. Rheumatol Phys Med 1970;suppl:88–92.

89. Huskisson EC. Measurement of pain. Lancet 1974;2:1127–31.

90. Hutchinson TA, Boyd NF, Feinstein AR. Scientific problems in clinical scales, as demonstrated in the Karnofsky index of performance status. J Chron Dis 1979;32:661–6.

91. Hutchinson TA, Flegel KM, Ho Ping Kong H et al. Reasons for disagreement in the standardized assessment of suspected adverse drug reactions. Clin Pharmacol Ther 1983;34:421–6.

92. Joint International Society and Federation of Cardiology/World Health Organization Task Force on Standardization of Clinical Nomenclature. Nomenclature and criteria for diagnosis of ischemic heart disease. Circulation 1979; 59:607–9.

93. Joyce CRB, Zutshi DW, Hrubes V, Mason RM. Comparison of fixed interval and visual analogue scales for rating chronic pain. Europ J Clin Pharmacol 1975;8:415–20.

94. Kalton G, Roberts J, Holt D. The effects of offering a middle response option with opinion questions. Statistician 1980;29:65–78.

95. Kane RA, Kane RL. Assessing the elderly: A practical guide to measurement. Lexington, MA: Lexington Books, DC Heath and Co, 1981.

96. Karnofsky DA, Burchenal JH. The clinical evaluation of chemotherapeutic agents in cancer. In: MacLeod CM, ed. Evaluation of chemotherapeutic agents. New York: Columbia Univ Press, 1949:191–205.

97. Kasl SV. When to welcome a new measure. Am J Public Health 1984;74:106–8.

98. Katz S, Ford AB, Moskowitz RW, Jackson BA, Jaffee MW. Studies of illness in the aged. The Index of ADL: A standardized measure of biological and psychosocial function. JAMA 1963;185:914–9.

99. Keele KD. The pain chart. Lancet 1948;2:6–8.

100. Keys A, Fidanza F, Karvonen MJ, Kimura N, Taylor HL. Indices of relative weight and obesity. J Chron Dis 1972;25:329–43.

101. Killip T, Kimball JT. Treatment of myocardial infarction in a coronary care unit. A two year experience with 250 patients. Am J Cardiol 1967;20:457–64.

102. Komaroff AL, Black WL, Flatley M, Knopp RH, Reiffen B, Sherman H. Protocols for physician assistants. Management of diabetes and hypertension. N Engl J Med 1974;290:307–12.

103. Komaroff AL, Ervin CT, Pass TM, Sherman H. Protocols in ambulatory care. Public Health Rev 1978;7:135–55.

104. Kraemer HC. Ramifications of a population model for k as a coefficient of reliability. Psychometrika 1979;44:461–72.

105. Kramer MS, Feinstein AR. Clinical biostatistics: LIV. The biostatistics of concordance. Clin Pharmacol Ther 1981;29:111–23.

106. Kramer MS, Barr RG, Leduc DG, Boisjoly C, Pless IB. Maternal psychological determinants of infant obesity. Development and testing of two new instruments. J Chron Dis 1983;36:329–35.

107. Kremer E, Atkinson JH, Ignelzi RJ. Measurement of pain: Patient preference does not confound pain measurement. Pain 1981;10:241–8.

108. Kuder GF, Richardson MW. The theory of the estimation of test reliability. Psychometrika 1937;2:151–60.

109. Landis RJ, Koch GG. The measurement of observer agreement for categorical data. Biometrics 1977;33:159–74.

110. Lansbury J. Quantitation of the activity of rheumatoid arthritis. 5. A method for summation of the systemic indices of rheumatoid activity. Am J Med Sci 1956;232:300–10.

111. Lansbury J. Report of a three-year study on the systemic and articular indexes in rheumatoid arthritis. Theoretic and clinical considerations. Arthritis Rheum 1958;1:505–22.

112. Likert R. A technique for the measurement of attitudes. Arch Psychol 1932;22:1–55.

113. Lindzey G, Aronson E, eds. The handbook of social psychology. Vol 2, 2nd ed. Reading: Addison-Wesley Publishing Co, 1968.

114. Littman GS, Walker BR, Schneider BE. Reassessment of verbal and visual analog ratings in analgesic studies. Clin Pharmacol Ther 1985;38:16–23.

115. McDermott W, Rogers DE. Technology's consort. Am J Med 1983;74:353–8.

116. McGuire RJ, Wright V. Statistical approach to indices of disease activity in rheumatoid arthritis. Ann Rheum Dis 1971;30:574–80.

117. MacKenzie CR, Charlson ME. Standards for the use of ordinal scales in clinical trials. Br Med J 1986;292:40–3.

118. Mahler DA, Weinberg DH, Wells CK, Feinstein AR. The measurement of dyspnea. Contents, interobserver agreement, and physiologic correlates of two new clinical indexes. Chest 1984;85:751–8.

119. Mahler DA, Matthay RA, Snyder PE, Wells CK, Loke J. Sustained-release theophylline reduces dyspnea in nonreversible obstructive airways disease. Am Rev Respir Dis 1985;131:22–5.

120. Mahoney FI, Barthel DW. Functional evaluation: The Barthel index. Md State Med J 1965;14:61–5.

121. Matthews DA, Feinstein AR. A "review of systems" for the personal aspects of patient care. Clin Res 1985;33:259A.

122. Meenan RF, Gertman PM, Mason JH. Measuring health status in arthritis. The Arthritis Impact Measurement Scales. Arthritis Rheum 1980;23:146–52.

123. Messick S. Test validity and the ethics of assessment. Am Psychol 1980; 35:1012–27.

124. Miller GA. The magical number seven, plus or minus two: Some limits on our capacity for processing information. Psychol Rev 1956;63:81–97.

125. National Diabetes Group. Classification and diagnosis of diabetes mellitus and other categories of glucose intolerance. Diabetes 1979;28:1039–57.

126. Norris RM, Brandt PWT, Caughey DE, Lee AJ, Scott PJ. A new coronary prognostic index. Lancet 1969;1:274–8.

127. Ohnhaus EE, Adler R. Methodological problems in the measurement of pain: A comparison between the verbal rating scale and the visual analogue scale. Pain 1975;1:379–84.

128. Oppenheim AN. Questionnaire design and attitude measurement. New York: Basic Books Inc, 1966.

129. Payne SLB. The art of asking questions. Princeton: Princeton Univ Press, 1951.

130. Peel AAF, Semple T, Wang I, Lancaster WM, Dall JLG. A coronary prognostic index for grading the severity of infarction. Brit Heart J 1962;24:745–60.

131. Peto R, Pike MC, Armitage P, Breslow NE, Cox DR, Howard SV, Mantel N, McPherson K, Peto J, Smith PG. Design and analysis of randomized clinical trials requiring prolonged observation of each patient. I. Introduction and design. Br J Cancer 1976;34:585–612.

132. Pincus T, Summey JA, Soraci SA Jr, Wallston KA, Hummon NP. Assessment of patient satisfaction in activities of daily living using a modified Standard Health Assessment Questionnaire. Arthritis Rheum 1983;26:1346–53.

133. Pozen MW, D'Agostino RB, Mitchell JB, Rosenfeld DM, Guglielmino JT, Schwartz ML, Teebagy N, Valentine JM, Hood WB Jr. The usefulness of a predictive instrument to reduce inappropriate admissions to the coronary care unit. Ann Intern Med 1980;92:238–42.

134. Pozen MW, D'Agostino RB, Selker HP, Sytkowski PA, Hood WB Jr. A predictive instrument to improve coronary-care-unit admission practices in

acute ischemic heart disease. A prospective multicenter clinical trial. N Engl J Med 1984;310:1273–8.

135. Ransohoff DF, Feinstein AR. Problems of spectrum and bias in evaluating the efficacy of diagnostic tests. N Engl J Med 1978;299:926–30.

136. Reger RB, Peterson MR, Morgan WKC. Variation in the interpretation of radiographic change in pulmonary disease. Lancet 1974;1:111–3.

137. Rose GA. The diagnosis of ischaemic heart pain and intermittent claudication in field surveys. Bull World Health Org 1962;27:645–58.

138. Sackett DL, Chambers LW, MacPherson AS, Goldsmith CH, McCauley RG. The development and application of indices of health: General methods and a summary of results. Am J Public Health 1977;67:423–8.

139. Sackett DL, Haynes RB, Tugwell P. Clinical epidemiology. A basic science for clinical medicine. Boston: Little, Brown, 1985.

140. Samet JM. A historical and epidemiologic perspective on respiratory symptoms questionnaires. Am J Epidemiol 1978;108:435–46.

141. Schachtel BP, Fillingim JM, Beiter DJ, Lane AC, Schwartz LA. Rating scales for analgesics in sore throat. Clin Pharmacol Ther 1984;36:151–6.

142. Scott J, Huskisson EC. Graphic representation of pain. Pain 1976;2:175–84.

143. Smythe HA, Helewa A, Goldsmith CH. "Independent assessor" and "Pooled index" as techniques for measuring treatment effects in rheumatoid arthritis. J Rheumatol 1977;4:144–52.

144. Sokal RR, Sneath PHA. Principles of numerical taxonomy. San Francisco: WH Freeman and Co, 1963.

145. Sonquist JA, Baker EL, Morgan JN. Searching for structure. An approach to analysis of substantial bodies of micro-data and documentation for a computer program. Ann Arbor: Survey Research Center, Institute for Social Research, The University of Michigan, 1973.

146. Spitzer RL, Chairperson, Task Force on Nomenclature and Statistics. Diagnostic and statistical manual of mental disorders. 3rd ed. Washington DC: American Psychiatric Association, 1980.

147. Spitzer WO, Dobson AJ, Hall J, Chesterman E, Levi J, Shepherd R, Battista RN, Catchlove BR. Measuring the quality of life of cancer patients: A concise QL-index for use by physicians. J Chron Dis 1981;34:585–97.

148. Sriwatanakul K, Kelvie W, Lasagna L, Calimlim JF, Weis OF, Mehta G. Studies with different types of visual analog scales for measurement of pain. Clin Pharmacol Ther 1983;34:234–9.

149. Stoller JK, Ferranti R, Feinstein AR. Further specification and evaluation of a new clinical index for dyspnea. Am Rev Respir Dis (In Press).

150. Teasdale G, Jennett B. Assessment of coma and impaired consciousness: A practical scale. Lancet 1974;2:81–4.

151. Thurstone LL, Chave EJ. The measurement of attitude. Chicago: Univ Chicago Press, 1929.

152. Torgerson WS. Theory and methods of scaling. New York: John Wiley and Sons, 1967.

153. Ware JE Jr, Brook RH, Davies AR, Lohr KN. Choosing measures of health status for individuals in general populations. Am J Public Health 1981;71:620–5.

154. Weinstein MC, Fineberg HV. Clinical decision analysis. Philadelphia: WB Saunders, 1980.
155. Wells CK, Feinstein AR, Walter SD. Comparison of predictive accuracy of multivariate models for survival in lung cancer. Clin Res 1985;33:268A.
156. Williams ME, Hadler NM, Earp JAL. Manual ability as a marker of dependency in geriatric women. J Chron Dis 1982;35:115–22.
157. Willoughby JMT, Kumar PJ, Beckett J, Dawson AM. Controlled trial of azathioprine in Crohn's disease. Lancet 1971;2:944–7.
158. Zyzanski SJ, Hulka BS, Cassel JC. Scale for the measurement of "satisfaction" with medical care: Modifications in content, format and scoring. Med Care 1974;12:611–20.

Index